A Team Approach to the Aquatic Continuum of Care

A Team Approach to the Aquatic Continuum of Care

Charlotte O. Norton, D.P.T., M.S., A.T.C., C.S.C.S.
Building Bridges Aquatic Consulting, Sacramento; Motion Analysis
Lab Physical Therapist, Shriners Hospitals for Children, Sacramento

Lynette J. Jamison, M.O.T., O.T.R./L
Owner, Future Waves: Aquatic Therapy Consultation, Phoenix;
Lymphedema Therapist, Phoenix

Foreword by
Bruce E. Becker, M.D.
Medical Director, St. Luke's Rehabilitation Institute, Spokane,
Washington; Clinical Associate Professor, Department of
Rehabilitation Medicine, University of Washington School of
Medicine, Seattle

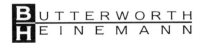

Boston   Oxford   Auckland   Johannesburg   Melbourne   New Delhi

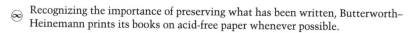
∞ Recognizing the importance of preserving what has been written, Butterworth–Heinemann prints its books on acid-free paper whenever possible.

 Butterworth–Heinemann supports the efforts of American Forests and the Global ReLeaf program in its campaign for the betterment of trees, forest, and our environment.

Library of Congress Cataloging-in-Publication Data
Norton, Charlotte O.
    A team approach to the aquatic continuum of care / Charlotte O. Norton, Lynette J. Jamison.
        p.   cm.
    Includes bibliographical references and index.
    ISBN 0-7506-7168-8 (alk. paper)
    1. Hydrotherapy—Practice. 2. Continuum of care. I. Jamison, Lynette. II. Title.
    [DNLM: 1. Hydrotherapy. 2. Continuity of Patient Care. 3. Patient Care Planning.
    4. Patient Care Team. WB 520 N883t 2000]
    RM811.N67 2000
    615.8'53--dc21

                                   99-058263

British Library Cataloging-in-Publication Data
A Catalogue record for this book is available from the British Library.

The publisher offers special discounts on bulk orders of this book.
For information, please contact:
Manager of Special Sales
Butterworth–Heinemann
225 Wildwood Avenue
Woburn, MA 01801-2041
Tel: 781-904-2500
Fax: 781-904-2620

For information on all B–H medical publications available, contact our World Wide Web home page at: http://www.bh.com

10 9 8 7 6 5 4 3 2 1

Printed in the United States of America

To my parents, Ada Bliss Norton and Frederick Minter Norton, who brought me here for this opportunity; to my lifelong mentors Russ Lauber, M.S., Laurie Stewart-Burns, M.S., P.T., and Gary L. Soderberg, Ph.D., P.T., F.A.P.T.A., who have inspired me to have a personal vision, work hard, and think beyond possibility; and to my dear friends and colleagues Helen Tilden and Dianne Rothhammer-Sheetz for their unrelenting love and support.

C.O.N.

Dedicated to my parents, Darleen and Jim Jamison, for their undying devotion; to my friends for their endless support; and to my aquatic staff, Nancy Kostura, Barbara Eccles, Peggy Santache, Susan Levesque, and Connie Sullivan, for their understanding and patience.

L.J.J.

Contents

Contributing Authors

Ellen Broach, Ph.D., C.T.R.S.
Assistant Professor, Department of Recreation
and Sports Management, Georgia Southern
University, Statesboro

Stacey DeGooyer, B.A., M.T.
Independent Massage Therapist, San Francisco

Ellen S. Garrison, M.Ed., R.K.T., A.T.R.I.C.
Aquatic Therapy Supervisor, Department
of Physical Therapy, Thoms Rehabilitation
Hospital, Asheville, North Carolina

Lynette J. Jamison, M.O.T., O.T.R./L.
Owner, Future Waves: Aquatic Therapy Consultation, Phoenix;
Lymphedema Therapist, Phoenix

Carol A. Kennedy, M.S.
Program Director Fitness/Wellness, Division of
Recreational Sports, Indiana University, Bloomington

Charlotte O. Norton, D.P.T., M.S., A.T.C., C.S.C.S.
Building Bridges Aquatic Consulting, Sacramento;
Motion Analysis Lab Physical Therapist, Shriners
Hospitals for Children, Sacramento

Fran Coffey Stanat, Ph.D.
Director, Therapeutic Recreation Program, School of Allied Health
Professions, University of Wisconsin, Milwaukee

Helen M. Tilden, R.N.
Director of Education, Building Bridges
Aquatic Consulting, Atlanta

Foreword

The international renaissance in aquatic therapy is well underway. Following a period of nearly 50 years during which the aquatic medium was used in only very limited ways in health management or restoration, aquatic rehabilitation has very strongly emerged once again into the mainstream of contemporary rehabilitation techniques. Twenty years ago, it was rare to find pools in therapy clinics. Today, most new facilities have included a pool as a valued and utilized feature. Contemporary hospitals have built pools to serve both inpatient and outpatient populations. Patient awareness of the value of the aquatic environment is at a high level; I rarely need to stress the potential value of aquatic rehabilitation to my patients to get them into the water, whereas several years ago, it was often a struggle.

This renaissance did not occur by chance. It was driven by a diverse group of aquatic believers, coming from a broad range of backgrounds. The growth of aquatic rehabilitation occurred through the efforts of many kinds of therapists: occupational, physical, recreational, kinisiotherapy, massage, as well as athletic trainers and exercise physiologists. I might humbly add that several physicians aided the cause as well. These diverse clinicians had seen the value of the aquatic environment in injury recovery, fitness development and maintenance, and health management; and they struggled to create new techniques or adapt established ones and proselytized colleagues to join the aquatic movement. It has taken nearly 20 years to achieve the current head of steam, to use an appropriately aquatic metaphor.

Much research has been done into the physical effects of the aquatic environment, extending over many years and body systems. Little of this research has been published within the rehabilitation or therapy literature but rather in the physiology literature or in medical subspecialty journals. But the science is very solid. Arguably, there is better scientific support for the use of the aquatic environment in rehabilitation and health maintenance than almost any other treatment technique. But the work is far from finished. The rehabilitation literature still lacks high-quality aquatic research studies. We do not know the best treatment techniques for most clinical problems, or the ideal water temperatures, or the optimum treatment duration, or the best program progression methods. We lack accurate outcomes measurement tools, and we must have objective assessment methodologies. To fill these large gaps will require the combined efforts of a great many individuals, trained in a variety of backgrounds, and working in concert. The research ideally should extend across the entire continuum of care, from early injury recovery through complex rehabilitation, into life-long health maintenance. Most of us "true believers" feel that aquatic techniques potentially add value to all of these needs.

To my knowledge this book is the first to address the relationships among the diverse group of professionals with an interest in aquatic therapy. Despite numerous examples of superb working relationships among the many concerned disciplines, there are examples where the relationships have been discordant. This discord serves neither the patient nor the concerned disciplines well. In proposing the Lyton model as a method of creating a care continuum, this book offers a creative structure for program development that potentially makes maximum use of the many unique areas of training of each of the various disciplines.

The aquatic medium offers potential benefit for a huge portion of the population, extending these benefits across the age span and health continuum. Because of the magnitude of the population capable of benefiting, no single discipline can have primary "authority" over aquatics, lest we leave out some potential human gain. This book offers a strategy for recruiting and coordinating all of us toward a common goal, working in collaboration and mutual respect. On this foundation, the necessary structure for future research can be built. Immersed in this environment of mutual respect and support, the health benefits of the aquatic medium can be extended across the population in need, which certainly includes ourselves, present and future.

Bruce E. Becker, M.D.

Preface

This book will provide the aquatic and rehabilitation fields with a multidisciplinary continuum of care to develop an integrated interdisciplinary treatment plan. The continuum of care will follow the acute phase of an illness, injury, or other surgical procedure through fitness to wellness. This book describes the skills and training of team members and how each contributes to a return to independence and a healthy, active lifestyle. Use of personnel is explained for all members of the rehabilitation team to maximize resources, increase productivity, improve clinical outcomes, and prevent consumer fraud.

The disciplines represented include occupational therapy, physical therapy, exercise physiology, athletic training, therapeutic recreation, kinesiotherapy, massage therapy, and fitness professionals. Each discipline in this book is represented by individuals who are recognized in the aquatic industry as experts. The authors were chosen for their knowledge both in aquatics and their respective field.

This book will provide physicians, case managers, educators, therapists, and nonlicensed personnel a resource for clear understanding of the appropriate level of referral and third party billing. The text will clearly describe the role of each discipline in the aquatic continuum of service to prevent misrepresentation of education, training, ability, or skills by nonlicensed personnel to the client or insurance company.

Chapter 1 has been written as an introduction to aquatic rehabilitation, fitness, and wellness. In Chapter 2, the Lyton model describes the aquatic continuum of care. Chapter 3 addresses licensure, certification, registration, and title acts. Chapter 4 was written to describe

training available for the various techniques utilized in aquatic rehabilitation. A chapter has been dedicated to each discipline involved in
aquatics to describe specific education and training and how each professional participates within the Lyton model. Finally, case studies are
included to help the reader understand each discipline's role in the
care of the client.

L.J.J.
C.O.N.

Acknowledgments

This book was a collaborative effort. All of the contributing authors labored over the development and revisions of their chapters. Each author was challenged to critically assess her role in the aquatic continuum of care. This was a difficult task because the nature of the project to define controversial boundaries can create turbulence within professional communities. A heartfelt thanks to each of the authors willing to take the risk and put their words on paper.

A special thanks to Lynette Jamison for working diligently to bring this project to fruition. Through the process of writing this book, our professional collegiality has bloomed into a friendship. Together we spent many hours working on this project. Through it all, maintaining our humorous perspectives made the unforeseen challenges manageable.

Lynette and I gratefully acknowledge Donna Andersen, P.T.A.; Anita Bagley, Ph.D.; Lori Thein Brody, M.S., P.T., S.C.S., A.T.C.; Ellen Epping, M.S., A.T.C.; Cheryl Fuller, A.T.C.; Kimberly Olsen, M.P.T., A.T.C.; Andrea P. Salzman, M.S., P.T.; Mary Sanders, M.S.; Helen Tilden, R.N.; and Debra Willardson, M.S., P.T., A.T.C., for their time reviewing the manuscript and providing feedback and encouragement.

My deepest appreciation to my family and special friends who have shared with me their warmth, compassion, love, and support during my many life endeavors, including this book. My relationships with all of you provide me with the strength to risk failure in order to succeed.

This book represents my belief that we all bring unique gifts to the water. We must work together to build bridges between the medical, fitness, and wellness communities to produce positive outcomes for those we serve. It is a tribute to all of the professionals in the aquatic world working to provide clients with the opportunity to move toward new levels of health and wellness.

C.O.N.

Aquatics and aquatic rehabilitation have been my life's interest. As a child, swimming and diving in the neighborhood pool was a way of life. Waterskiing during summer vacations at Lake Powell, Page, Arizona, is and always will be one of my fondest memories. Learning to scuba dive as a young adult was a logical progression in my aquatics interests. Spending long weekends on the Pacific Ocean scuba diving off the Channel Islands gave me a love of water that would be unsurpassed. A scuba dive master once said to me during one of our ocean outings, "you should have a career doing what you love to do." In choosing a career, the words "doing what you love to do" influenced my decision to become an aquatic occupational therapist.

In 1989, I became the director of an outpatient aquatic center and maintained that position through mid-1999. During those years, my staff and I became Watsu® practitioners and received training from multiple sources, including the Aquatic Therapy Symposium sponsored by the Aquatic Therapy Rehabilitation Institute, Arthritis Foundation, United States Water Fitness Association, and the American Red Cross. Our facility was recognized as having Excellence in Innovations, by the Arizona Hospital Association, for our aquatic programming for patients and community members. The United States Water Fitness Association recognized our facility from 1991 through 1997 as The Top Health Institute Aquatic Program in the United States for our programs, staff credentials, and sponsored educational courses. We were able to host annual continuing education courses such as aquatic Feldenkrais®, Watsu®, aquatic proprioceptive neuromuscular facilitation (PNF), Arthritis Foundation/YMCA aquatic program instructor courses, and American Red Cross water safety classes.

This manuscript is my effort to define the roles of the different allied health professionals who provide aquatic services in order to preserve our positions in the aquatics industry. Only through communication, education, and understanding of the aquatic industry can we move forward in a pro-active fashion and embrace the essence and power of the aquatic medium.

I extend my deepest gratitude to my loyal aquatic staff for their undying efforts to continually improve the services at our facility. Their courage during the untimely closure of our pool gave me the strength to go forward and complete this manuscript.

Recognition is in order to those who have assisted the process of writing this book. Charlotte and I give our appreciation to Connie Sullivan; David Ogden, P.T.; Karen Bowen O.T.R./L; and Ruth Meyer, R.K.T., for their editing efforts. Their editorial comments were invaluable. Marcia Lorona and Julie Hedelson have provided tremendous transcript, clerical, and editorial support in the final days of this manuscript. Their efforts were tireless. A special thanks to Chris Oagley, Lisa Quinn, and Troy Sorrells for their creativity in developing the graphics for this text.

My mother, Darleen Jamison, has given of herself to me and has given me guidance with her wisdom and strength.

Charlotte O. Norton has been supportive to me with her gentle strength and hilarious sense of humor. Charlotte and I made the decision to produce a book that would provide the aquatics industry with a guide to the roles of aquatic disciplines. Without Charlotte, this book might not have been written.

L.J.J.

CHAPTER 1

Introduction

Lynette J. Jamison and Charlotte O. Norton

Water is the essential fluid for life. Ancient cultures considered hot springs to be divine and water was used in religious rituals for purification.[1,2] The use of water for therapeutic purposes is documented since the time of ancient Greece.[1] The word *hydrotherapy* is Greek in origin: *hydro* means "water," and therapeia means "healing." Hippocrates referred to the use of water for muscle and joint disorders.[2] Greek athletes received water treatments for rehabilitation. The Romans were aware of the beneficial effects of mineral water and built large thermal baths with pools of water at different temperatures.[2] The remains of these complexes may be seen today in the English town of Bath.[1]

Balneotherapy further developed in Europe. In Germany, warm baths were used to relax muscle spasms; in England, cold baths were used to treat conditions of fever. In the 19th century, physicians scientifically studied the physiological responses to immersion in water of different temperatures, and the medical benefits of water treatments were established.

In the United States, hydrotherapy was developed as a treatment modality for neurologic rehabilitation, initially in response to the polio epidemic, and following World War I, as treatment for amputees.[2,3] Further research into the effects of water immersion resulted from National Aeronautics and Space Administration (NASA) experiments designed to simulate reduced gravity environments. Today in the United States, the term *hydrotherapy* commonly is used to describe the use of whirlpools to cleanse wounds. Since the early 1980s, American therapists have used the term *aquatic therapy* to describe the rehabilitation process in water. Applications of aquatic therapy are expanding rapidly and populations treated include those with neurologic, orthopedic, and rheumatic conditions and those with sports injuries.

The interest in aquatic therapy has exploded in the United States. Aquatic services are provided by a full spectrum of professionals, from a licensed physical or occupational therapist to an aquatic guru who has many years of practical application in water activity. Aquatic therapy has become a multidisciplinary field. Each professional's role in the world of water has not been clearly defined, and this has created confusion for consumers, payers, and providers.

In 1996, the American Physical Therapy Association's (APTA) Aquatic Physical Therapy Section drafted a document proposing standards to guide physical therapists practicing therapy in the water. The recommendations for basic clinical competencies address patient care skills, interpretation of examination findings and assessment, and designing integrated land-pool treatment programs into the physical therapy plan of care. Daily pool operations, program administration, and evaluation also are addressed within the draft document developed by the APTA aquatic section (see Appendix A).[4]

In 1996, the Aquatic Therapy Rehabilitation Institute (ATRI) (see Appendix A) recognized the need to develop a set of standards to assist the many professionals involved in aquatic wellness and rehabilitative services. These standards provide guidelines that assist in defining aquatic therapy and wellness practice in the water. The standards are written in general terms to accommodate multiple settings and multiple disciplines. In 1998, the ATRI established a multidisciplinary aquatic therapy certification to provide credentials for those who successfully indicate minimum competency and knowledge in aquatic rehabilitation and wellness.

The challenges in defining aquatic rehabilitation stem from the differences in education and individual state practice acts for each professional who treat clients in the water. Our contention is that aquatic rehabilitation is completed by a continuum of therapy, fitness, and wellness. The term *rehabilitation* in its broadest sense means restoration of or return to ability. In 1947, the National Council on Rehabilitation defined rehabilitation as "the restoration of the handicapped to the fullest physical, mental, social, vocational, and economic usefulness of which they are capable."[5] The term *habilitation* was used to describe children who were not developed and were born with or acquired disability shortly after birth.[5] Today, *habilitation* is extended to indicate improvement of functioning beyond any previous condition.

The terms *rehabilitation* and *habilitation* derive the complex philosophy that the total capabilities of each patient must be considered. The licensed practitioner must consider an individual's life components when a program of care is designed, because disabilities interfere with one's capability to live a full life. Therefore, appropriate interventions must be implemented for a return to a better quality of life. More than 50 years after the National Council on Rehabilitation defined *rehabilitation*, therapists use aquatic rehabilitative therapy for a return to a better quality of life in all components.[5]

Fitness is defined (in *Webster's Encyclopedic Unabridged Dictionary of the English Language*) as the state of being in good physical conditioning thereby indicating good health. *Aquatic fitness* may refer to general condition exercises including cardiovascular, aerobic, strengthening, toning, range of motion, and flexibility activities.

Wellness can be described as the integration of health and behavior to be "well" even in the presence of illness or disease.[5] A state of wellness reduces the risk of illness and disease, providing satisfaction, control, and the ability to do more and take interest in the future. It is a concept that evolved during the mid-1900s as Americans, especially women and members of minority groups, became disenchanted with the medical practices and attitudes of clinicians.

The Lyton model for the aquatic continuum of care refers to a range of services available in the water. The goals for these services are to improve life's components in keeping with true rehabilitation. The continuum presents a wide range of specific services for specific outcomes. The client may enter the continuum at any phase of the model. The entry level is dictated by the level of illness, wellness, and needs or goals of each individual. These goals may be general fitness, stress reduction, and special needs, such as those following polio or one-on-one therapy for recovery.

Aquatic therapy training is not a consistent standard or base of any curriculum in the rehabilitation disciplines, such as physical therapy, occupational therapy, recreational therapy, and kinesiotherapy. Therefore, those who receive aquatic rehabilitative training must seek courses following graduation. Many courses in aquatic therapy and therapeutic techniques are not restricted to licensed physical and occupational therapists and few are offered at the university level.

The information, techniques, and education of aquatic rehabilitative trainers varies. For example, some instructors may have adequate skill with the Halliwick method of aquatic technique but may not understand disease pathology of a particular client. Or the therapist may have adequate skill in land-based therapeutic exercise and not understand hydrophysics. Aquatic education providers have various levels of knowledge related to disease pathology and aquatic rehabilitation principles. The result of this type of education at best is unpredictable.

Nonlicensed practitioners, such as exercise physiologists, adaptive aquatic specialists, and aquatic fitness instructors, may or may not possess certification from organizations such as America College of Sports Medicine (ACSM), Aquatic Exercise Association (AEA), International Dance Education Association (IDEA), United States Water Fitness Association (USWFA), or the YMCA. The purpose of such certification is to ensure a safe land, water fitness, aerobic, or exercise class, not provide rehabilitative therapy. There is no provision of disease pathology in an aquatic fitness instructor's training.

The delivery of services and their outcome vary when assessment, treatment, and documentation are not uniformly administered. The Lyton model (see Chapter 2) was developed as an aquatic continuum of care to offer a clear delineation of aquatic service providers and as a definition of the continuum of rehabilitative care within the context of aquatic services commensurate with education and training.

With the circular Lyton model, there is no hierarchical chain of care. The method provides an entry at the appropriate level for rehabilitation following an injury, wellness, or overall fitness. With this method, a service delivery plan to meet each person's individual needs easily is accomplished in an economical, time-efficient manner. For example, an athlete has different needs than an older adult with arthritis. The athlete wants a quick return to competition, the person with arthritis wants to remain independent, mobile, and free from pain. The programs differ and the level of education and skill also differs to meet the service delivery to each person. In addition to physical and occupational therapy, other services in the Lyton model include relaxation for wellness, independent specific home exercise program (HEP), and special population groups, with each member of the team contributing to components of the client's life.

Relaxation for wellness may include services such as Watsu® water massage or Ai Chi (water Tai Chi). Today's alternative medicine supports taking care of oneself from a holistic perspective by reducing stress. Warm water is innate to stress reduction with the support of buoyancy and the warmth of a therapeutic pool.

An independent specific HEP contain exercises given to a client by a licensed therapist to be used during and after the client has completed a regime of one-on-one treatment. The exercises are designed to augment and enhance the therapy. The general purpose of a HEP is to aid in the continued progress of a client.

Special group programs are aquatic exercise classes for those with special needs such as arthritis, recovery from polio, multiple sclerosis, fibromyalgia, back injury, or traumatic brain injury. In general, the individuals who participate in these classes have needs which could be provided in groups of four or more. The services provided may improve cardiovascular fitness, strength, range of motion and flexibility, overall fitness for independent living, socialization, and psychosocial support.

One-to-one aquatic therapy is provided by licensed therapists. Clients who require one-on-one aquatic therapy have medical complications that require specific assessment and treatment. If treated by individuals who lack medical knowledge, serious consequences could occur, such as reinjury or exacerbation of the condition.

References

1. Skinner AT, Thomson AM. *Duffield's Exercise in Water*. London: Bailliere Tindall; 1983:4–198.
2. Ruoti RG, Morris DM, Cole AJ. *Aquatic Rehabilitation*. Philadelphia: Lippincott; 1997:3–402.
3. Becker BE, Cole AJ. *Comprehensive Aquatic Therapy*. Boston: Butterworth–Heinemann; 1998:1–177.
4. Aquatic Physical Therapy Section. *Basic Clinical Competencies Draft 3*. Fairhope, AL: PRADCOM; February 1998.
5. Hopkins HL, Smith HD. *Willard and Spackman's Occupational Therapy*, 6th ed. Philadelphia: J.B. Lippincott; 1983:3–24.

CHAPTER 2

The Lyton Model for the Aquatic Continuum of Care

Charlotte O. Norton and Lynette J. Jamison

The Lyton model depicts the aquatic continuum of care (Figure 2–1). The client is in the center of the model to illustrate the importance of consequences in decision making. All services and referrals using the Lyton model focus on the client.

The triangle represents licensed treatment, fitness, and wellness. Licensed treatment in this model is provided by professionals who maintain a license to practice in a particular state. Licensed professionals are held accountable for following their state practice act guidelines. Medicare states that reimbursable therapy services must be provided by a practitioner who maintains a license.

Fitness refers to an apparently healthy[1] client working toward a state of physical well being as determined by measures such as VO_2 max. The professional working with this individual will have a specialized background in water fitness. Wellness in the Lyton model refers to the client who has a chronic disease, such as arthritis, and is trying to improve the quality of his or her life through the use of an aquatic medium. The professional working in the wellness arena also must have specialized training in water exercises for those with special needs.

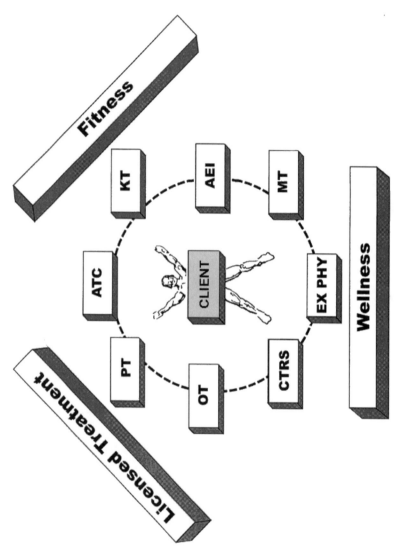

FIGURE 2–1.   Lyton model depicting the aquatic continuum of care.

Each professional working in the water is placed along an *iso-chronal* line in a circle indicating movement within the continuum. The circle eliminates the hierarchical structure and provides an opportunity for the client to receive the appropriate care in the aquatic environment through referrals.

The case studies that follow demonstrate the application of the Lyton model for the aquatic continuum. Information is provided to assist the clinician in understanding the client from a global perspective. The range of motion (ROM) measures assume the client is able to start at the anatomical position or neutral unless otherwise noted. Several manual muscle-testing scales are available to measure strength. The grade 3/5 indicates full range of movement against gravity. Grades of 1 and 2 indicate that the client is unable to actively move against gravity. This client should be placed in a position or environment that reduces gravitational forces. Grades of 4 and 5 indicate the client has full range of movement against moderate and maximal resistance respectively. Occasionally, dynamometer measurements are available that allow the clinician to calculate the amount of torque the client is able to generate. Dynamometry, if applied correctly, offers a more quantifiable measure of strength; however, it is not as widely used in the clinical setting.

These case studies are based on actual clients with some modifications to illustrate the continuum of care. Not every discipline is appropriate to work with every type of client. For example, athletic trainers do not work with clients who have had a cerebrovascular accident because this pathology is not a component of their education and training.

The goals were developed by each discipline on the basis that humans function on land; however, the water is the tool used to achieve the goals. The case study about Roxanna has been integrated into the chapter of each discipline.

Roxanna (Diagnosis: Arthritis/Total Joint)

Social and Medical History

Roxanna is a 64-year-old woman with a combination of osteoarthritis and rheumatoid arthritis. She weighs 205 pounds and is 5 feet tall. The initial diagnosis of arthritis was made at age 43. She was told she would need to lose weight and exercise three to five days per week. At age 56, Roxanna fell, broke her right hip, and received a total hip replacement.

Roxanna lives in a ground-level house with her mother. They share the household responsibilities and grocery shopping. Roxanna finished the twelfth grade by taking special education classes. Her intellectual level is slightly impaired. She reads at the sixth grade level.

Current Medical Status

Roxanna is currently experiencing an exacerbation of rheumatoid arthritis. She has a perceived pain level of 7/10 (0 indicates no pain).

Medications

She is taking an anti-inflammatory and a medication for pain.

Exam Findings

Range of motion: Active right hip flexion 90° without pain, left hip flexion 80° with increased pain at end range of available motion. Right knee flexion 80°, left knee flexion 75°, ankle dorsiflexion limited to neutral and painful. Trunk rotation was painful and within functional limits. Shoulder flexion was 130° bilaterally. Elbow flexion was within functional limits. Wrist and fingers were limited and painful with an ulnar deviation observed.

Strength: Upper extremity strength 3/5, trunk strength 3/5, hip flexion 2+/5.

Sensation: Sensation was within normal limits throughout the upper and lower extremities, trunk, hands and feet.

Mobility/function: Roxanna demonstrates a bilateral Trendelenberg gait pattern. Roxanna ambulates with a wheeled walker during exacerbation of her arthritis. Transfers from sitting to standing are difficult and standby assistance is necessary for bath bench transfers; however, she is independent. She uses a step-to-gait pattern for ascending and descending stairs. She demonstrates appropriate hip precautions for limited right hip flexion, adduction, and internal rotation.

Activities of daily living: Roxanna is able to bathe and dress while sitting using adaptive devices. Maximum assistance is necessary for heavy household chores, such as vacuuming and cleaning the shower.

Leisure Assessment

Roxanna lives a sedentary life. Prior to her hip replacement, she enjoyed water aerobics. She feels the pain and her weight are barriers to her participation in leisure activities. She also demonstrates the depression and low self-esteem associated with chronic pain.

Fitness Assessment

Roxanna's mobility has been limited by pain, therefore her overall endurance is very limited.

Resting heart rate: 75 bpm.

Blood pressure: 138/88.

Body composition: 39% body fat.

Discipline-Specific Goals

OT: Roxanna will transfer on and off a shower bench independently and will increase participation with household chores to include vacuuming a 10 × 10 foot area.

PT: Roxanna will strengthen bilateral hip abductors to minimize her Trendelenberg gait when she returns to walking without an assistive device. She also will demonstrate improved upper and lower extremity strength to increase the ease of sit-to-stand transfers.

TR: Roxanna will maintain her strength and abilities in water activity, transfers into the water, and comfort in the water to facilitate future leisure involvement in an arthritis aquatic program for pain reduction and weight loss.

EP: Roxanna will reduce her body fat by ½% per month. She will understand how to exercise using the Borg Rate of Perceived Exertion scale.

MT: Roxanna will experience decreased pain and increased range of motion.

ATC/AEI/KT

Roxanna will participate in an arthritis aquatic program three times per week to increase or maintain her mobility and encourage socialization.

Application of the Lyton Model

Roxanna entered the model after her total hip replacement, to be seen by the PT and OT to address problems in range of motion, strength, gait, transfer between sitting and standing, and activities of daily living. Once discharged from an inpatient setting, Roxanna may continue with outpatient PT and OT services to achieve her goals. Depending on the facility, an exercise physiologist may address issues related to body composition and exercise intensity for cardiovascular endurance. She may also see a CTRS to address her leisure goals. Once discharged from an outpatient setting, Roxanna may be enrolled in an arthritis aquatic program taught by any of the professionals in the Lyton model, with proper education, including KT, AEI, and MT.

Roxanna may move throughout the Lyton model during different times in her life. She may require PT and OT during exacerbation of her rheumatoid arthritis. Changes in her recreational activities and cardiovascular fitness may require additional input from the CTRS and EP. The other professionals in the Lyton model continue to play an active role in Roxanna's wellness by providing opportunities for decreased pain and maintenance of mobility and function.

James (Diagnosis: C6 Incomplete SCI)

Social and Medical History

James is a 45-year-old man, 6 feet, 4 inches tall, weighing 240 pounds. James is married and his wife appears very supportive. He smokes three cigars per day. Prior to the injury, James worked as a sales representative for computer software company. He currently works four hours per day from his home. His right hand is dominant.

In a motor vehicle accident four months ago, he suffered an incomplete spinal cord injury at C6. He had a fusion of the C5 and C6 vertebrae. He also suffered a fracture in the midshaft of his right humerus, which was immobilized for six weeks. He underwent intensive inpatient therapy (occupational, physical, and recreational) for 10 weeks. He has been in outpatient therapy for the past six weeks.

Current Medical Status

James has stabilized medically. X rays show the fusion demonstrates good bone growth and the humerus is healed. He continues to show improvement in functional strength and mobility, including ambulation on all surfaces with a single axis cane. James continues to demonstrate residual deficits in balance and truck control for gross motor activities. He has difficulty with range of motion and grip strength in his right hand. He is right-handed and has difficulty performing fine motor coordination tasks such as shaving and brushing his teeth. Handwriting is possible but difficult to read.

Medications

Neurotonin.

Exam Findings

Range of motion: Upper extremities and lower extremities are within functional limits with the exception of the right shoulder, active abduction 0–110°, flexion 0–114°, external rotation 0–33°.

Strength (manual muscle testing): Sitting—hip flexion R 4–/5, L 4/5; knee flexion R 4–/5, L 4/5; extension R 4/5, L 4/5; ankle dorsiflexion R 4/5, L 4/5; plantarflexion R 4+/5, L 4+/5; shoulder flexion R 3+/5, L 4/5; abduction R 3+/5, L 4–/5; elbow flexion R 4–/5, L 4/5; extension R 3+/5, L 4/5. Prone—hip extension R 4+/5, L 4/5; internal rotation R 4/5, L 4+/5; external rotation R 4+/5, L 4+/5. Sidelying—hip abduction R 3+/5, L 4–/5; adduction R 3/5, L 2+/5. Jamar dynamometer grip strength in kilograms force R 36, L 65.

Sensation: Intact to light touch and sharp/dull in bilateral upper and lower extremities.

Mobility/function: James demonstrates caution with all transfers including supine to sitting, sitting to supine, and sitting to standing. James requires two to three attempts to move from sitting to standing. He initially pauses for 3–5 seconds and shifts his feet to gain his balance using a single axis cane. James can perform static single leg stance on the right 11 seconds, left leg 15 seconds without loss of balance (normal estimated at 25–30 seconds). Tinetti balance and gait 15/28, which places him at high risk for falls (balance 11/16; gait 4/12 with a single axis cane). Get up and Go test 37.5 seconds.

Activities of daily living: James is independent in gross motor activities such as bathing, washing his hair, and donning T-shirts and sweatpants. He has mild difficulty manipulating buttons and shoelaces. He continues to experience some difficulty with balance when putting away dishes or carrying books from the den to his computer desk.

Leisure Assessment

Prior to his accident, James enjoyed motorcycling and golf. He wants to return to these activities. Jack also stated an interest in learning to become independent in swimming and water skiing so he could continue participation in enjoyable pursuits that are challenging and healthy.

Fitness Assessment

James's overall level of fitness is poor. While he has been active during his lifetime, his recreational pursuits have not included any aerobic activity. He demonstrates some shortness of breath with increased exertion.

Resting heart rate: 70 bpm.

Blood pressure: 130/84.

Discipline-Specific Goals

OT: James will improve fine motor coordination to allow independence in manipulating buttons and shoelaces as he dons slacks, dress shirts, and tennis shoes. He will demonstrate strategies and adaptive techniques to safely carry dishes to the kitchen sink and his books for 10 feet.

PT: James will safely ambulate up to 50 feet without the use of an assistive device. He will demonstrate a heel-to-toe gait pattern for distances longer than 50 feet using a single axis cane. His Tinetti balance and gait score will be 22/28, and his Get up and Go test score will improve to 13 seconds.

TR: James will become independent in planning community outings and report comfort in public by discharge. James will develop the skills to participate in golf (a preinjury interest) and develop skills for independent participation in water activity to meet his motivational needs of challenge, maintenance of physical ability, and social interaction.

EP: After participating in a submaximal bike test, James's fitness level will be assessed and the MET level for aerobic activity determined. His low level of fitness will be considered to progress his aerobic activity to ensure an enjoyable experience. His blood pressure will be monitored during and after aerobic activity to ensure an appropriate response.

MT: James will demonstrate increased range of motion. The MT will facilitate relaxation to stimulate the body's healing system.

ATC: James will return to a golf program when released from therapy.

AEI: James will begin water walking classes and progress to aqua aerobics classes to increase endurance. Classes will include exercises for posture and body mechanics for sitting, standing, and walking. He will maintain a weekly workout with an aquatic personal trainer to practice skills for golf, such as posture, stance, swing, and follow through. Water jogging or aqua aerobics will be incorporated into the training program for cardiovascular endurance. The AEI will refer James to the EP to develop a personal workout if his schedule does not permit a regular workout with the personal trainer or AEI.

KT: James will demonstrate improvement in fitness parameters by report of perceived increase in functional endurance at home. James will learn a low-level endurance exercise in the water such as prone endurance with use of mask and snorkel.

Application of the Lyton Model

James entered the model as an inpatient after his spinal cord injury was stabilized. He was seen by the PT, OT, and TR to address problems in range of motion, strength, balance, gait, activities of daily living, and recreational interests. When discharged, James continued OT and PT as an outpatient to achieve his ambulation and ADL goals. Depending on the facility, James may be involved with community outreach recreational endeavors to address his leisure goals and KT to provide him fitness education. When discharged from outpatient therapy, James may be enrolled in an aquatic fitness program taught by any of the professionals in the Lyton model including KT, AEI, and MT.

James may move throughout the Lyton model during different times in his life. He may require PT if new injuries occur. He also may require EP for continued progression of strength and overall fitness education. The other professionals in the Lyton model provide opportunities for fitness, recreation and leisure interests, exercise, and maintenance of mobility and function.

George (Diagnosis: Cerebrovascular Accident with Right Hemiparesis)

Social and Medical History

George is a 69-year-old man, 6 feet, 2 inches tall, weighing 220 pounds. He had an embolitic cerebrovascular accident (CVA) seven days ago. Prior to the CVA, George lived with his wife of 40 years in their home. He is right-handed. Four steps with railings on both sides flank the entrance into the house. A bedroom and bathroom are on the first floor. The bathroom has no adaptive devices. His wife and daughter appear very supportive and want to take George home.

Past Medical History

HTN, L THA, hyperlipidemia, glaucoma.

Current Medical Status

George has moderate fluent expressive aphasia with minimal receptive comprehension. His speech consists mostly of jargon with consistent and appropriate yes and no answers. He has difficulty with mobility and transfers secondary to the right hemiparesis. Moderate to maximum assistance is necessary for bathing, dressing, and fine motor coordination activities such as shaving and brushing his teeth. His visual field is limited to the left side with no right-sided gaze, suggesting a right-sided neglect.

Medications

Heparin, Lopressor, Zoloft, Timpoptic Ophth, enteric-coated ASA, Docusate Na+, Nifedipine, Maalox.

Exam Findings

Range of motion: Passive range of motion within functional limits bilaterally for upper extremity and lower extremity. Right upper extremity is flaccid. Right hip internal rotators have increased activity with motion. Active range of motion within functional limits for left upper extremity and lower extremity and absent in right upper extremity and lower extremity.

Strength: Manual muscle test not completed due to patient's inability to follow commands for holding against resistance on today's date.

Sensation: Patient responded to painful stimuli bilaterally on upper extremity and lower extremity.

Mobility/function: Bed mobility—requires moderate assistance and verbal cueing with all bed mobility. Static sitting balance—able to sit unsupported for 3 minutes. Dynamic sitting balance—maintained while using left upper extremity to reach 6–12 inches for objects placed above and below shoulder level on the left side and below shoulder level on the right. He was unable to reach above shoulder level on the right and required a visual tracking cue to cross the midline. Experienced loss of balance once, reaching down and across midline to right. George had difficulty with standing due to right leg not extending to provide support. All transfers need maximum assistance by one person. He is able to take four small steps with a hemi-walker and moderate assistance by two people.

Activities of daily living: George is unable to balance while standing at the sink to brush his teeth and shave. He can brush his teeth while sitting supported, after a physical demonstration, using his left hand, however. Shaving was possible using an electric razor, after a physical demonstration, while sitting supported. He requires moderate assistance with donning sweatpants and T-shirts while reclining in bed. George can feed himself finger food using his left hand. He has difficulty using utensils.

Leisure Assessment

George's previous recreational interests included walking with his wife and playing basketball one time per week. George's wife wishes to learn an enjoyable activity they can pursue together during their free time. The family also wishes to learn to become comfortable transporting George in the family car to community activities.

Fitness Assessment

Resting heart rate: 66 bpm.

Resting blood pressure: 136/86.

Heart rate following ambulation of 10 feet: 78 bpm.

Blood pressure following exercise: 140/86.

Discipline-Specific Goals

OT: George will don T-shirts and sweatpants using an adaptive technique with standby and minimal assistance. He will groom and feed himself while sitting upright with setup assistance. He will attend to objects right of midline. George will perform right upper extremity weight-bearing exercises with setup and moderate assistance to minimize incidence of right shoulder subluxation.

PT: George will demonstrate improved right upper and lower extremity strength for increased ability to perform transfers. He will be independent in bed mobility. George will require minimal assistance of one person for all transfers. He will ambulate with a narrow-based quad cane on level and unlevel surfaces with minimal assistance. He will ascend and descend four stairs with railing and minimal assistance.

TR: George will participate in simple card games using a card rack. George will attend two community family training outings (one dinner outing and one outing of family choice). Family will report comfort in public before discharge.

EP: George will begin with 5 minutes of water walking to regain stability. Buoyant devices will be used to increase his stability walking in a gravity-reduced environment. Water walking will be increased in intensity and time to increase endurance and return George to the activity he enjoys with his wife, walking. Water walking time will be increased 5–10% per week based on his vital signs and perceived exertion. His blood pressure, heart rate, and rate of perceived exertion will be measured before, during, and after the activity. He will progress to 15 minutes of continuous walking in the pool. When this goal is achieved, he will begin treadmill walking (on land).

MT: Facilitate the movement of the right side of the body, release the tension of the left side of the body.

ATC: None.

AEI: George will advance to an arthritis aquatics class or "seniors" class for low-intensity exercises to maintain or increase range of motion of all joints and strengthen the musculoskeletal and cardiovascualar systems. The social atmosphere of the class and verbal games will provide an opportunity to use his tongue and palate and practice speech patterns.

KT: George will demonstrate improved standing balance and gait activities in pool.

Application of the Lyton Model

George entered the model after his CVA as an inpatient in an acute hospital setting to be seen by the speech language pathologist (not included in the Lyton model), PT, and OT to address problems in cognition and language, range of motion, strength, right-sided function, balance, gait, and activities of daily living. When medically stable, he will be transferred to a rehabilitation hospital for 14 days. Therapeutic recreation was integrated into his care plan. On discharge, he continued PT and OT as an outpatient.

George may be referred to community outreach programs to address his leisure goals. The EP and KT will provide fitness education.

Following discharge, George may be enrolled in an aquatic fitness program taught by any of the professionals in the Lyton model including KT, AEI, and MT.

George may move throughout the Lyton model during different times in his life. He may require PT and OT in times of status change, such as a painful right shoulder from subluxation. He also may require EP, KT, or AEI for continued progress in strength and overall fitness education. The other professionals in the Lyton model contribute to provide opportunities for fitness, recreation and leisure interests, exercise, and maintenance of mobility and function.

Curtis (Diagnosis: Anterior Cruciate Repair)

Social and Medical History

Curtis is a 19-year-old man, 5 feet, 11 inches tall, weighing 175 pounds. A collegiate skier at the University of New Hampshire, he was competing in Europe when he lost control on a jump and landed with his right knee hyperextended. Patient denies any significant prior medical history.

Current Medical Status

An MRI revealed a torn anterior cruciate ligament (ACL) and a small medial meniscus tear on Curtis's right knee. Surgical repair was completed using an autograft from the central third of his patellar tendon. A partial medial meniscectomy was also performed. Curtis is seen two weeks post-op in an outpatient evaluation. Sutures have been removed and the incision is healed.

Medications

Tylenol with codeine for pain.

Exam Findings

Range of motion: Active—hip and ankle within functional limits bilaterally, knee extension to flexion right 0–89°, left 2–0–135°.

Strength: Manual muscle test—bilateral hip, ankle and left knee 5/5; right knee extension and flexion not tested.

Sensation: Intact to light touch over bilateral lower extremities.

Mobility/function: Patient is independent in all activities of daily living. He currently has 50% of weight-bearing ability using two crutches.

Activities of daily living: He has difficulty putting on his right shoe and is otherwise independent.

Leisure Assessment

Curtis skis competitively at the collegiate level. He also enjoys playing basketball with his friend. He wants to continue preinjury activities.

Fitness Assessment

Curtis is in excellent physical condition. He would like to maintain this during his rehabilitation.

Discipline-Specific Goals

OT: Curtis will don his right shoe independently using a long shoehorn and elastic shoelace.

PT: Curtis will increase active range of motion and strength to allow him to return to skiing. He will demonstrate 90% or better ability for quadriceps and hamstrings isokinetic strength compared to his left knee.

TR: Curtis will increase active range of motion and strength to facilitate a return to preinjury activities of interest. Curtis will attend one community outing to address independence in community mobility and function. Curtis will develop skills in safe skiing and basketball technique.

EP: Curtis is in excellent shape. The challenge to the EP is maintenance of his fitness level during rehabilitation. We will focus on upper body strengthening activities in deep water. Deep water is chosen until full weight bearing is permitted and tolerated. We will use surface area devices, such as hand paddles, for overload to the upper body and trunk stablizers to increase overload and keep his upper body strong and trunk stabilizers while he heals. We also will introduce a land arm ergometer workout for 20 minutes, progressing to 60 minutes, to maintain upper body strength.

MT: Curtis will maintain agility in other areas of his body and release compensation muscles, reduce tightness in the quadriceps, hamstrings, and calf muscle.

ATC: Curtis will increase active range of motion and strength to allow him to return to skiing. He will demonstrate 90% or better quadricep and hamstring isokinetic strength compared to his left knee. He will maintain his cardiovascular endurance throughout the rehab process. Curtis will pass sports-specific testing to clear him for participation in competitive skiing.

AEI: Curtis will work with an aquatic personal trainer to perform simulated ski movements. Additional sports-specific movement patterns and plyometric exercises such as hops, jumps, and speed-reaction drills will be introduced. He will add deep water jogging as an adjunct to his training schedule.

KT: Same as ATC.

Application of the Lyton Model

Curtis entered the model after his knee injury as an inpatient in an acute hospital setting for surgery and to be seen by PT to address problems in range of motion, strength, and gait. The OT provided Curtis with a long shoehorn and elastic shoelaces and instructions for their use. Following discharge, he continued with the PT and ATC as an outpatient for skills to return to skiing. After discharge, he continued outpatient PT and ATC services to achieve his goals. Depending on the facility, Curtis may be involved with ATC directly following surgery for athletic retraining and EP to provide him with fitness education. Once discharged to an outpatient setting, Curtis may be involved with the ATC for return to skiing.

Curtis may move throughout the Lyton model during different times in his life. He may require consultation from one or more of the disciplines in times of health status change, such as a painful right knee, or reinjury.

Susie (Diagnosis: Cerebral Palsy with Spastic Right Hemiparesis)

Social and Medical History

Susie is a 14-year-old girl, 5 feet, 3 inches tall, weighing 96 pounds. Susie has problems related to independence, body image, acceptance. She is very self-conscious. She refuses to perform extracurricular activities due to the self-consciousness and fears failure. She also refuses to perform treatment activities. This limits development of performance skills, especially execution of motor movement, which in turn would increase her self-esteem.

Current Medical Status

Susie currently is medically stable. She has difficulty with general motor control due to the spasticity on the right side of her body.

Medications

Baclofen.

Exam Findings

Range of motion: Passive right shoulder flexion 0–145°; abduction 0–150°; internal rotation 0–30°; external rotation 0–45°. Active flexion of left shoulder, elbow, and wrist within functional limits. Passive right hip abduction 0–10°; flexion 0–94°; internal rotation 0–35°; external rotation 0–5°. Active flexion of left hip, knee, and ankle within functional limits. Posturing of right upper extremity in shoulder adduction, internal rotation, elbow flexion, and wrist flexion. Limitation in active movement of the right shoulder in flexion, abduction, rotation. Tends to flex, adduct, and internally rotate right hip during stance and ambulation.

Strength: Not tested due to patient's refusal.

Sensation: Poor kinesthetic sense on the right side of her body.

Mobility/function: Decreased functional use and decreased coordination of the right upper extremity during activities. Delayed balance and equilibrium responses. Left hand is dominant. No reciprocal arm swing in gait; right arm is held in a postured position.

Activities of daily living: Susie requires minimal assistance for donning blouses and slacks using her left upper extremity. Moderate assistance is necessary for donning socks and shoes. Susie can feed and groom herself using her left hand.

Leisure Assessment

Susie reports she wants to learn how to swim but lacks comfort swimming with others in public.

Fitness Assessment

Not done at this time.

Discipline-Specific Goals

OT: Susie will increase active and passive range of motion of the right shoulder. She will demonstrate increased functional use and coordination of the right upper extremity during bilateral activities. She will increase bilateral integration of her body during activities, especially those that involve balance and equilibrium. Achievement of goals will promote a positive self-image.

PT: Susie will increase active and passive range of motion of left hip for increased independence with mobility. Susie will independently ambulate 30–60 feet on a level surface safely with no assistive device. Susie will ride a stationary bike for 10 minutes with a resistance of 2.

TR: Susie will achieve the following swimming goals—increased bilateral movement and coordination of extremities, increased reciprocal movement of upper extremities, enhanced balance and equilibrium skills, providing a medium to heighten self-esteem.

EP: Utilize water exercise to develop muscular strength and endurance to prepare for swimming lessons and increase comfort in the water. Basic major muscle group exercises will be performed using surface area devices to increase endurance and strength. Other devices will be introduced to ensure an enjoyable experience.

MT: Have fun, build confidence, and facilitate a sensation of relaxation particularly of the right muscle groups.

ATC: None.

AEI: Find an aquatic instructor experienced in working with children. Use a buoyant cuff to increase kinesthetic awareness. Include low intensity exercises and static stretching to increase range of motion in shoulders, elbows, and wrist. Progress to a group class with other children to increase socialization. If instructor is a swimming instructor, add swimming lessons. It may be necessary to refer to a member of the team who is an adapted swimming instructor.

KT: Susie will demonstrate increased exercise capability, independence, and self-esteem while in the pool by learning an adapted swim position with appropriate floatation.

Application of the Lyton Model

Susie entered the model when she was born with cerebral palsy (CP). She has been treated by OT and PT for range of motion and mobility during her physical and mental developmental stages. She works with the CTRS to develop recreational activities that encourage social integration. The MT works with Susie to assist with relaxation. The EP provides Susie the opportunity to improve her overall fitness. The KT can provide education and fitness opportunities.

Susie will move throughout the Lyton model during different times in her life. She may require PT and OT when changes develop in mobility. Changes in her recreational activities and cardiovascular fitness may require additional input from the CTRS and EP. The other professionals in the Lyton model continue to play an active role in Susie's wellness by providing opportunities for maintenance of mobility and function and socialization with water activities.

Karen (Diagnosis: Multiple Sclerosis)

Social and Medical History

Karen is a 57-year-old woman, 5 feet, 1 inch tall, weighing 195 pounds. She initially was diagnosed with multiple sclerosis (MS) at the age of 42. She is experiencing difficulty with walking and urinary incontinence. She has no other significant medical history. She lives with her husband and reports she is independent in most activities of daily life. She does complain that she fatigues easily.

Current Medical Status

Karen walks with a front-wheeled walker. She is able to ambulate short distances (up to 15 feet) without her walker. She has had episodes of ataxia and recently fell and was unable to get up from the floor.

Medications

Prednisone, Baclofen.

Exam Findings

Range of motion: Active range of motion within functional limits bilaterally for upper extremity and lower extremity with the exception of her hip flexors, right 0–92°, left 0–87°.

Strength: Manual muscle test—upper extremity grossly 4/5 except left shoulder flexion 4–/5. lower extremity grossly 4–/5 bilaterally except for right knee flexion 4/5.

Sensation: Intact to light touch over bilateral upper extremity and lower extremity.

Mobility/function: Karen is independent in bed mobility and transfers. She ambulates up to 100 feet with front-wheeled walker before requiring a rest.

Activities of daily living: Karen is independent in her self-care. She bathes using cool water while sitting on a shower chair. She sits while donning slacks, socks, and shoes with some difficulty. She is responsible for meal preparation but requires frequent rest periods to complete tasks. Karen and her husband share the household chores. Karen becomes easily fatigued while cleaning the house.

Leisure Assessment

Karen reports she enjoys bowling but finds herself tiring easily. She is not sure that she wants to use adapted equipment to continue this activity. However, she stated that she wants to pursue activities that assist in maintaining her physical ability and social support and gives her a reason to get out of bed in the morning.

Fitness Assessment

Karen fatigues easily with all activities.

Resting heart rate: 76 bpm.

Blood pressure: 134/84.

Body composition: 41% body fat.

Discipline-Specific Goals

OT: Karen will demonstrate energy conservation techniques for performing activities of daily living including meal preparation and household chores. She will don socks and shoes using a long shoehorn and adaptive technique.

PT: Karen will ambulate 300 feet with front-wheeled walker before experiencing enough fatigue to require her to sit. To improve strength and mobility, Karen will demonstrate an appropriate intensity during an aquatic exercise program. Karen will verbalize understanding of heat and overactivity that causes fatigue and their effects on MS symptoms.

TR: Karen will participate in an MS aquatic program. Karen will demonstrate the ability to assess her fatigue level. Karen will explore local transportation options to attend class prior to discharge from TR. Arrange transportation to class prior to discharge. To facilitate continued participation Karen and her family will attend an outing with the therapist at the local MS aquatic exercise class for an orientation introduction to the facility and the aquatic exercise program.

EP: We will set specific body composition goals of a reduction of ½% body fat per month along with an increase in lean body weight. We also will monitor Karen's heart rate, blood pressure, and rate of perceived exertion throughout the aerobic exercise sessions for appropriate progressions.

MT: Create a sense of support and fluidity in the water and freedom from muscle noncooperation to practice gait patterns used on land. Walking in shallow water to provide tactile and proprioceptive input.

ATC: Client will participate in an MS aquatic exercise class three times per week to increase endurance.

AEI: MS aquatic classes to focus on balance and coordination and the socialization of a group setting. She will use buoyant equipment such as a bar float for ambulation and progress to resistive exercises to increase upper extremity strength using buoyant barbells. Limit use of bands or tubing that may bruise or tear the skin. She also will perform exercises to increase strength of hip flexors, ankle dorsiflexors, and hamstrings.

KT: Karen will demonstrate improvement in functional endurance by self-report of home activities. She will demonstrate the proper technique, safety measures, and ability to pace herself with a low-level endurance activity in the water, such as bicycling.

Application of the Lyton Model

Karen entered the model at the wellness level, where she engaged in aquatic exercises supported and sponsored by the National Multiple Sclerosis Society. After class one day, the AEI noticed that Karen had difficulty with balance and donning her socks and shoes. The AEI suggested that Karen see her doctor for the possible need of OT and PT. Karen followed up with her doctor and was referred to the OT and PT. The OT provided Karen a long shoehorn and elastic shoelaces and instructed her in their use. The OT also provided education and energy conservation techniques, including a home visit to adapt the kitchen, laundry room, and other areas for activities of daily living. The PT worked with Karen to develop improved dynamic balance to allow her to successfully continue participation in classes taught by the AEI. She may also see the MT or CTRS if relaxation and recreation issues need to be addressed.

Karen may move throughout the Lyton model during different times in her life. She may require services from various disciplines in times of status change or exacerbation of her MS.

Jack (Diagnosis: Lumbar Fusion)

Social and Medical History

Jack is a 33-year-old, white, married man, who reported pain in his lower back and a lower extremity radiculopathy. Jack, an attorney who enjoys playing golf, lives with his wife and two daughters.

Current Medical Status

He was diagnosed by MRI with degenerative disk disease in his lumbar spine with some instability, which was thought to be causing his pain. He underwent an anterior lumbar fusion, L4 to S1. Now at six weeks post-op, he continues to report pain along the right L4 dermatome. He has not returned to work, because it requires sitting for four hour periods and standing for long periods of time during court proceedings. The courthouse has long hallways and walking is painful.

Medications

None.

Exam Findings

Range of motion: Active trunk range of motion limited by 75% in all directions in standing, hip, knee, and ankle within functional limits bilaterally. Hamstring length measured in supine position with hip and knee in 90° of flexion right –35°, left –40°.

Strength: Manual muscle test: hip abductors 3/5 bilaterally, flexion and extension 4/5 bilaterally, knee and ankle 4+/5 bilaterally for all motion.

Sensation: Intact to light touch. Some hypersensitivity noted in the right L4 dermatome. Patellar tendon and Achilles tendon reflexes intact and symmetrical.

Mobility/function: Bilateral Trendelenberg gait. Ambulating without an assistive device.

Activities of daily living: Jack is independent. He reports some difficulty putting on his shoes and socks. He is unable to sit for longer than 1 hour and therefore unable to return to work.

Leisure Assessment

Jack enjoys playing golf and participating in family activities.

Fitness Assessment

Previously, Jack had not exercised regularly. He is not familiar with how to monitor his heart rate.

Discipline-Specific Goals

OT: Jack will demonstrate proper joint protection techniques and body mechanics related to performing his job and self-care. He will use adaptive techniques to don his socks and shoes.

PT: Jack will demonstrate increased trunk and lower extremity range of motion per protocol to allow ease with activities of daily living. Jack will demonstrate increased hip abductor strength to prevent antalgic gait patterns.

EP: Jack will participate in a submaximal exercise test to establish a baseline of aerobic fitness. We will introduce Borg rate of perceived exertion with the chart of 6–20. A heart rate monitor will be utilized to equate the "feeling" to a number on the Borg scale. During this test we also will teach Jack about heart rate training. We will utilize a heart rate monitor to teach him how it "feels" to be at a certain heart rate level. We will establish a target heart rate and introduce deep-water exercise with a focus on functional movements for a return to the game of golf. We will set target heart rate goals for him and encourage him to try deep-water exercise with a focus on functional movements so he can get back to his golf.

MT: Jack will be provided with modified Watsu® to reduce pain in his lower back and leg.

ATC: Jack will demonstrate increased tolerance to sitting for 4 hours while doing computer work for a return to work. Jack will participate in return to work program including back care education.

AEI: Jack will begin with water walking classes and progress to aqua aerobics classes to increase endurance. Classes will include exercises for posture and body mechanics for sitting, standing, and walking.

He will maintain a weekly workout with an aquatic personal trainer to practice skills for the game of golf such as posture, stance, swing, and follow through with water jogging for cardiovascular endurance. Refer to EP to develop a personal workout if his schedule on return to work does not permit a routine workout with a personal trainer.

KT: Jack will demonstrate increased trunk stability and conditioning by a gradual progression of stabilization exercise.

Application of the Lyton Model

Jack started seeing a physical therapist when he hurt his back. In addition to his land-based treatment, he was referred to an aquatic back class instructed by an EP. After Jack's condition did not improve, he was referred back to the physician. He underwent a surgical fusion. While in the hospital he was assessed by PT and OT to address range of motion, strength, gait, and transfer training and activities of daily living. Once discharged from inpatient care, Jack continued outpatient PT services to achieve his goals. Depending on the facility, an exercise physiologist may address issues related to body composition and exercise intensity for cardiovascular endurance. Jack also saw a CTRS to address his leisure goals. Following discharge from outpatient therapy, he was referred to a return-to-work program coordinated by the ATC to resume work without limitations. Following the return-to-work program Jack indicated his increased interest in maintaining his improved health. He was referred to an AEI with specialized training for post-rehabilitation conditioning to develop a program to meet his fitness goals. He may also be seen for by the MT for Watsu® to promote relaxation and stress management.

Jack may move throughout the Lyton model during different times in his life. He may require PT and OT during exacerbation of his back pain. Changes in his recreational activities and cardiovascular fitness may require additional input from the EP or AEI. All professionals in the Lyton model continue to play an active role in Jack's wellness by providing opportunities for maintenance of mobility and function.

Reference

1. American College of Sports Medicine. *ACSM's Guidelines for Graded Exercise Testing and Prescription,* 5th ed. Baltimore: Williams and Wilkins; 1995.

CHAPTER 3

Licensure, Registration, Certification, and Title Acts

Lynette J. Jamison

Proving competency in the medical field usually is based on obtaining registration, various forms of certification, and often a medical or an allied health license. Physicians, nurses, physical therapists, occupational therapists—all are examples of medical professionals who become "licensed" to do their work. Many of these professions have set standards of practice that outline very specifically the privileges and limitations of practitioners.[1]

The medical profession generally is regulated by the state or jurisdiction. The jurisdictions include the 50 United States, Puerto Rico, District of Columbia, and the Virgin Islands. State regulation and national certification are different.[2]

The primary function of state regulation is to provide consumer safety and public protection. Most states require a minimum competency for licensure of all physicians and most allied health care providers. States regulate all health care and allied health care licenses.

A state license grants a practitioner permission to practice in that jurisdiction. States that license allied health professionals prohibit unlicensed individuals from practicing a licensed therapy or using that therapy's title. Regulatory requirements vary from state to state and from discipline to discipline. State boards also have the power to enforce discipline of a licensed practitioner.[3]

National certification protects the title of the practitioner and prohibits noncertified individuals from calling themselves by a given practitioner's title. In most cases, national certification requires passing a test and with an acceptable score. Most states and jurisdictions require national certification before they will issue a state license.[3]

The Continuum of Regulation

Four categories of state or national regulation may be designated in a continuum, from most to least regulated: licensure, certification, registration, and title acts or trademark laws.[3] There is, however, conflict regarding the continuum of regulation and their definitions. For example, the National Board for Certification in Occupational Therapy (NBCOT) offers the title of Occupational Therapist Registered to occupational therapists and certification to occupational therapy assistants for the title of Certified Occupational Therapy Assistant (COTA). Registration and certification in this instance are regarded equally regulated by the NBCOT.

Licensure always is state regulated and provides the highest quality of protection for the consumer by defining scope of practice and holding therapists accountable for their professional conduct. The scope of practice gives detailed rules and standards to which a practitioner legally must adhere. Note that a state regulatory agency can take action against a therapist's license. The licensed therapist can be warned. The license may be suspended or revoked for the following infractions: providing services outside the practitioner's scope of practice, unethical conduct, or malpractice. A license may be obtained after graduation from an accredited college or university program, completion of the required internship, successfully passing a license examination, and proper completion of the license application. For example, for an occupational therapist to receive a license in Arizona, she or he must demonstrate successful completion of an accredited occupational therapy program, the required six months of fieldwork, and a passing score on the certification examination sponsored by NBCOT.[3-5]

Certification is offered by state and national organizations. In most cases, certification provides a comprehensive definition of the discipline including explanation of scope of practice. Disciplinary action may or may not be included as part of the certification. In the case of physical therapy, the states and jurisdictions have coordinated national certification with state licensure with the Federation of State Boards for Physical Therapy (FSBPT). In this instance each state is responsible for the scope of practice and disciplinary action. Each state's physical therapy scope of practice is individual, however, it is supported directly by the American Physical Therapy Association (APTA).

Certification may be achieved after graduation from an accredited college or university program, completion of the required internship, successfully passing a certification examination, and proper completion of the certification application.[3-5]

Registration also can be sponsored by state or national organizations. Registration may or may not offer a defined scope of practice and disciplinary action. Registration is obtained after graduation from an accredited college or university program, successfully passing a registration examination, and proper completion of the registration application.[3-5]

Title acts and trademark laws basically entitle one to practice after graduation from an accredited college or university program. No formal application is required, no regulatory agency monitors conduct, and no disciplinary action can be taken. People who have not graduated from an allied health program may call themselves therapists; however, facilities will not employ persons without supporting education.[5]

Licensure offers consumer protection through a disciplinary action process. Certification and registration may or may not offer a disciplinary action process. Each discipline is regulated differently. A therapist does not have a choice which form of regulation they obtain. Regulation is discipline specific. Athletic trainers, for example, are nationally regulated with certification whereas occupational therapists are regulated through state licensure and national certification.

Program Certification

Program certification provides health and fitness professionals with public recognition of their knowledge, technical skills, and experience in a particular field or specialty. It certifies that the individual is qualified to practice in accordance with the standards deemed essential by the certifying body.[6,7] Program certification is documentation to provide this status and specify qualification. Exercise physiologists, for example, are certified by the American College of Sports Medicine (ACSM) to provide cardiac rehabilitation. ACSM certification is nationally recognized. Reimbursement from insurance companies, health maintenance organizations (HMOs), and third-party payers for cardiac rehabilitation services is state dependent.[8]

Occupational, physical, and recreational therapists and kinesiotherapists are required to take a national certification exam. This ensures neither state licensure nor third-party, HMO, or Medicare reimbursement. Practitioners must apply separately for a state license in each discipline. The national certification provides the state information regarding the applicant's qualifications.

State regulation (license), national certification, and national registration are different. A state license grants permission to a practitioner to practice in a particular jurisdiction. Requirements vary among the jurisdictions.[2]

Regulation by Profession

Aquatic Exercise Instructor

The fitness profession has no standard level of competency. Several land and aquatic fitness organizations offer certification for learning a given protocol. For example, the Arthritis Foundation joined with the YMCA to create Arthritis Foundation YMCA Aquatic Program (AFYAP). This program certifies the instructor to teach the arthritis aquatic program. There is no prerequisite for attending the course. In other words, the student instructor could be simply a high school graduate.

Athletic Trainer

Certification by the National Athletic Trainers Association (NATA) Board of Certification provides national recognition that an athletic trainer has met several professional requirements, including

- Successful completion of an accredited baccalaureate athletic training program.
- 800 contact hours supervised by an Athletic Trainer Certified (ATC).

- A passing score on the NATA certification examination.
- Eight continuing education units every three years.

Certification also can be obtained through an internship program by taking fewer required core courses at the college or university level and completing 1500 supervised hours. However, NATA recently established new criteria that will eliminate the internship option for certification in the year 2004.

Thirty-nine states regulate athletic training. Twenty-one states require licenses for ATCs, eight states require certification, six states require registration, and four states have exemptions. Texas established its own certification procedure. Although the remaining 11 states recognize national certification, it is not regulated.

Recreational Therapist

Certification by the National Council on Therapeutic Recreation Certification (NCTRC) provides national recognition that a practitioner has met several professional requirements, including

- Successful completion of an accredited baccalaureate therapeutic recreation program.
- Completion of 10 weeks of internship.
- A passing score on the NCTRC examination.
- Completion of 50 continuing education units every five years.

South Carolina and Utah are the only states that require certified therapeutic recreation specialists (CTRS) to be licensed. California has a practice act that limits the use of the title and defines the scope of practice.[9]

Exercise Physiologist

Exercise physiologists need no national certification. Louisiana is the only state to license exercise physiologists. Almost all practicing exercise physiologists have at least one certification through the American College of Sports Medicine. There are established prerequisites for the ACSM certifications. Within the ACSM clinical track, the exercise specialist certification requires a baccalaureate degree in an allied health field and a minimum of 600 hours of fieldwork in a clinical exercise program.

Within the ACSM health fitness track, the health fitness specialist certification requires educational training equivalent to an undergraduate or graduate degree in a health and fitness curriculum and the successful completion of a written and practical examination.

The majority of exercise physiologists who work in the clinical setting are trained at the graduate level and have worked specifically in exercise physiology. It has been estimated that more than 600 organizations offer some form of certification for exercise physiologists.[10] Unfortunately, prior education may not be necessary for anyone attending these certification courses.

According to Rosche,[11] insurance in the United States will pay for treatment of diseases diagnosed by health care professionals licensed to practice within their particular states. There has been some discussion at the American College of Sports Medicine national meetings concerning the pros and cons of licensure of exercise physiologists. Currently, several states are considering licensure but only for the clinical exercise physiologist.[12]

In July 1995, the Louisiana state legislature passed a bill (Senate Bill 597) regulating clinical exercise physiologists. The bill primarily sets the scope of practice for cardiac rehab services, but issues such as weight management, diabetes, and cancer are listed within the text. One would think that, with licensure, Louisiana exercise physiologists automatically would get reimbursed through insurance and third-party payers, but this has not been the case. Several clinics have reported that they have not increased third-party billing due to this change. We are learning from Louisiana that licensure does not guarantee reimbursement. However, Louisiana may ensure the clinical exercise physiologist's place in the medical field at a later date, even though it is not happening now.

Kinesiotherapist

Registration by the American Kinesiotherapy Association (AKTA) provides national recognition that a kinesiotherapist (KT) has met certain professional requirements, including

- Successful completion of a baccalaureate accredited kinesiotherapy program.

- Completion of 1000 hours of clinical training.
- A passing score on the AKTA written and practical certification examination.
- Completion of 50 continuing education units every three years.

Only three states recognize the profession of kinesiotherapy: New Hampshire, Ohio, and Virginia. As a result, KTs often practice as nonlicensed aides under the direction of a physical therapist.[13]

Massage Therapist

In the United States, massage regulation is inconsistent. No government oversight is provided at the national level. Only Washington, D.C., and 24 of the 50 states currently have laws requiring some form of licensure, certification or registration. Twenty-one states are regulated, four states have passed laws that are not yet in effect, and one state has regulation in process.[14] State laws supersede local regulations, yet many city and county government agencies do not want to relinquish the regulation of massage. The result is wide discrepancy in the laws, ordinances, rules, and regulations governing massage therapy from one locality to the next.

Where licensing is available, the prevailing trend is toward requiring a 500-hour curriculum. There is much controversy regarding the scope of practice and other issues. For example, in Louisiana, physical therapists are working to keep licensed massage therapists from performing neuromuscular therapy and other techniques prescribed by a doctor. Under Wisconsin's registration law, a massage therapist can practice if the terms *massage* or *bodywork* are not used. Several professional massage organizations are self-regulating bodies that maintain registries and referral programs. These organizations provide continuing education and offer technique-specific certification. They discipline massage therapists by revoking certification. They include the Worldwide Aquatic Bodywork Association (WABA), Aquatic Bodywork International (ABI), Jahara Technique Central Office, American Massage Therapy Association (AMTA), Associated Bodywork and Massage Professionals (ABMP), International Massage Association (IMA), American Oriental Bodywork Therapy Association (AOBTA), National Certification Board for Therapeutic Massage and Bodywork (NCBTMB).

Occupational Therapist

Certification by the National Board for Certification in Occupational Therapy (NBCOT) provides national recognition that an occupational therapist (OT) has met certain professional requirements, including

- Successful completion of an accredited masters of occupational therapy program.
- Completion of six months of field work.
- A passing score on the NBCOT certification examination.
- Completion of a renewal application every fifth year.
- Documentation of completion of required continuing education hours.
- The individual's attestation of good character.

Forty-one states require licenses for occupational therapists. To qualify for a state license, the OT must furnish documentation for all of the requirements of certification by NBCOT and every one to two years complete the renewal application, which includes documentation of continuing education requirements. Continuing education requirements vary from state to state, as do renewal applications.[15]

In addition to the states that require licenses, three states require certification: Vermont, Wisconsin, and Indiana. Four states require registration: Hawaii, Minnesota, North Dakota, and South Carolina. A total of forty-nine states provide regulation in the form of licensure, certification, or regulation of occupational therapists. Colorado has no regulation for OTs.[15]

Certified Occupational Therapy Assistant

Certification by the National Board for Certification in Occupational Therapy provides national recognition that a certified occupational therapy assistant (COTA) has met certain professional requirements, including

- Successful completion of an accredited COTA program.
- Completion of 440 hours or twelve weeks of field work.
- A passing score on the NBCOT certification examination for COTAs.

The occupational therapy assistant provides support to the occupational therapist and must work under the supervision and direction of the OT. Several states license occupational therapy assistants and require the successful completion of the NBCOT exam.[15]

Physical Therapist

Certification by the FSBPT provides national recognition that a physical therapist (PT) has met certain professional requirements, including

- Successful completion of an accredited baccalaureate physical therapy program.
- A passing score on the national physical therapy licensure examination.
- Completion of required internship.

Fifty-three states and jurisdictions require licenses for physical therapists. To qualify for a state or jurisdictional license the PT must furnish documentation of all the requirements of certification by the APTA and every year or two years complete the renewal application, which includes documentation of continuing education requirements. Continuing education requirements vary from state to state, as do renewal applications.[2, 16,17]

Physical Therapy Assistant

The physical therapy assistant (PTA) is a graduate of a two-year associates degree program. Certification by the FSBPT provides national recognition that a PTA has met certain professional requirements, including

- Successful completion of an accredited PTA program.
- Completion of three two-week affiliations and three eight-week internships.
- A passing score on the national physical therapy assistant exam.

The physical therapy assistant provides support to and must work under the supervision and direction of a physical therapist.

Several states license physical therapy assistants and require the successful completion of the NPTA exam. Forty-three states regulate PTAs, while forty-six states have title protection. Thirty-three states license PTAs, five states certify PTAs, five states register PTAs.[2, 16,17]

References

1. National Organization for Competency Assurance. What NOCA does. Available at: www.noca.org. Accessed July 1999.
2. American Physical Therapy Association. *State Licensure Reference Guide.* Alexandria, VA: APTA; July 1998 (revised).
3. Schmitt K, Shimberg B. *Demystifying Occupational and Professional Regulation: Answers to Questions You May Have Been Afraid to Ask.* Lexington, KY: Council on Licensure, Enforcement and Regulation; 1996.
4. Counsel on Licensure, Enforcement and Regulation. About CLEAR. Available at: www.clearhq.org. Accessed July 1999.
5. Interprofessional Workgroup on Health Professionals Regulation. Views on the licensure and regulation of health care professionals. Available at: www.ncsbn.org. Accessed November 1996.
6. Neiman D. *Exercise Testing and Prescription, a Health Related Approach.* Mountain View, CA: Mayfield Publishing; 1999:66–69.
7. Peterson JA, Bryant CX, Stevenson R. Making professional certification work for your facility. *Fitness Management.* July 1996:36–38.
8. American College of Sports Medicine. *ACSM's Guidelines for Graded Exercise Testing and Prescription*, 5th ed. Baltimore: William and Wilkins; 1995.
9. American Therapeutic Recreation Association. Standards for the practice. Available at: www.atra-tr.org. Accessed June 1999.
10. DuBois PC. Certification: How to spot the real thing. *Fitness Management.* August 1995:46–48.
11. Roche C. *The Insurance Reimbursement Manual for America's Body Workers, Body Therapists, and Massage Professionals*, 2nd ed. Cupertino, CA: Bodytherapy Business Institute; 1991.
12. Durak E, Shapiro A. *The Ins and Outs of Medical Insurance Billing*, 2nd ed. Santa Barbara, CA: Medical Health and Fitness Publication; 1996.
13. American Kinesiotherapy Association. Accreditation, education and training. Available at: www.akta.org. Accessed 1999.
14. U.S. law and legislation. *Massage Magazine.* 1999;79:134–135.

15. National Board for Certification in Occupational Therapy. What we do. Available at: www.nbcot.org. Accessed July 1999.
16. American Physical Therapy Association. Licensure examination candidate resources. Available at: www.apta.org. Accessed July 1999.
17. Federation of State Boards of Physical Therapy. Directory of state boards. Available at: www.fsbpt.org. Accessed June 1999.

CHAPTER 4

Aquatic Rehabilitation Techniques and Education

Lynette J. Jamison and Charlotte O. Norton

Hydrotherapy has enjoyed a long and well-chronicled history through the ages. Hot and cold baths were used to treat disease as far back as 460 B.C. In Europe almost 300 years ago, hot water was used with patients who were spastic or had muscle spasms and cold water was used to reduce fevers. During the late 1700s, cold water was being used for the treatment and comfort of smallpox victims.[1]

By 1830, Vincent Pressnitz combined cold water with a vigorous exercise program to strengthen patients who were ill. Pressnitz's work stimulated considerable thought in Europe; and for the first time, scientific investigation was done to test the reaction of tissues to water at various temperatures and their reaction time in disease. Dr. Winterwitz of Vienna, Austria, took part in these investigations and continued to research the effects of water at different temperatures on sick patients, eventually establishing an accepted physiological basis for hydrotherapy that still stands. Various states of rejuvenation through water may very well be linked to the fact that the human body is 98% water.[1]

Today, therapeutic aquatic exercise is used to effectively treat arthritis, multiple sclerosis, rheumatism, musculoskeletal problems, neurologic problems, cardiopulmonary pathology, and other conditions.[2] Although aquatic exercise may not cure these problems completely, it promotes strength, increased mobility and flexibility, improved circulation and relaxation.

The risks of aquatic rehabilitation and exercise are minimal. The primary risk of aquatic activity is drowning. According to the American Red Cross, the three most prevalent causes of drowning in pools are (1) hazardous conditions and practices, such as diving in shallow water; (2) inability to get out of dangerous situations; and (3) lack of knowledge about the safest ways to aid a drowning person. Training in basic water safety skills can prevent drowning.[3] The secondary risk of exercising in water, whether therapeutic or aerobic, is overdoing it. Because of water's buoyancy, an individual may not recognize the level of intensity being exerted. Risks may exist for those who are diabetic since overexercising can cause a rapid insulin uptake.

Hydrodynamic Principles Utilized During Aquatic Activities

Hydrodynamic principles such as buoyancy, temperature, hydrostatic pressure, viscosity, turbulence, and surface tension are incorporated into aquatic treatment to enhance the treatment program. Aquatic professionals should have knowledge of the properties and characteristics of water.

Buoyancy

The tremendous advantage of water exercise lies in buoyancy. Buoyancy provides support. The buoyancy of the water minimizes the effects of gravity, allowing support for painful joints and assistance for weak muscles.[4] Since buoyancy offsets gravity, an individual can change his or her experience of weight simply by moving to deeper water. A person waist deep in the water may experience approximately 50% of his or her weight while being chest deep equates to 25–30%. However, a person who is neck deep experiences only about 10% of his or her weight.[2] This support allows people who are overweight or have painful joints, particularly in the knees and hips, to exercise safely and pain free in water. In fact, impact can be completely eliminated by using flotation devices when exercisers are in deep water. Many excellent programs are available for exercising in deep water as well as in water that is waist or chest high. These programs are effective in improving fitness, strength, and flexibility for healthy persons as well as for those with injuries and disabilities.

Temperature

Therapeutic exercise usually takes place in warm water (approximately 90–94°), and exercise takes place in tepid water (approximately 84–90°) in depths ranging from 2 to 10 feet. The support and warmth of the water actually decreases pain and muscle spasms, which allows the patient an increased range of motion, strength, and relaxation. In addition, warm water next to the skin and muscles may cause the superficial blood vessels to dilate, thereby increasing circulation. The heart rate decreases in warm and tepid water and then increases proportionately to the intensity of exercise. Therefore, in comparison with other forms of exercise, a greater level of exercise may be tolerated in water while maintaining a lower heart rate and producing a decrease in pain.[2,5]

Hydrostatic Pressure

Hydrostatic pressure profoundly affects the cardiovascular, respiratory and nervous systems. Hydrostatic pressure is the multidimensional pressure applied to a body immersed in a fluid. The deeper the immersion, the greater the pressure. The effects of hydrostatic pressure occur the moment a person enters the pool.

Cardiovascular System

When a person is immersed in water, hydrostatic pressure forces blood from the legs into the chest. The heart fills with this excess blood, causing the heart muscle to stretch. When the heart muscle is stretched, it produces an increased muscle contraction, causing it to empty more completely. This is called *Starling's law.* Starling's law results in fewer heartbeats per minute to pump the same volume of blood. Therefore, immersion in water improves the efficiency of the heart muscle.[2,5-7]

Renal System

The renal system maintains the amount of fluid in the human body at a constant level. The hypothalamus in the brain measures fluids in the body. When a body is immersed in water, it is engorged with blood, and the brain interprets this as the body being overhydrated. To eliminate the excess fluid, the body senses a need to urinate. Once out of the water, the excess blood leaves the brain, and this is interpreted by the hypothalamus as being underhydrated and, therefore, the person feels thirsty.[2,5-7]

Respiratory System

With immersion in water, hydrostatic pressure forces blood from the legs into the chest. Blood engorges the lungs, making it harder to breathe. Additionally, the weight of water on the outside of the chest puts pressure on the diaphragm. The weight of water on the chest causes resistance to the diaphragm with breathing and forces air out of the lungs.[2,5-7]

Nervous System

The nervous system interprets information about the body's position in space, temperature, pressure, and sensation. When immersed in water, the body receives sensory information about water pressure and temperature. Immersion in water decreases pain due to oversensory stimulation. In a sense, the body is being bombarded with sensation.[2,5-7]

A major clinical application of immersion is to reduce edema. Immersion reduces edema more rapidly than bed rest and has the additional benefits of active exercise. Immersion exercises for women who are pregnant offer several advantages over land-based exercise. Buoyancy allows pregnant women to exercise without causing injury to weight-bearing joints while supporting the fetus, taking strain from the lower back. Hydrostatic pressure assists in the production of amniotic fluid, and warm water increases circulation to the muscles.

Viscosity

Viscosity refers to the thickness and stickiness of a liquid. Viscosity provides resistance to movement. Moving in water in any direction is resistive. The viscosity of warm water in a pool is less than cold seawater. Viscosity is the quality that makes water a useful strengthening medium, because it resists more as more force is exerted against it. However, the resistance stops instantly when the force ceases. As a result, when a client who is rehabilitating feels pain and stops movement, the force drops instantly, which allows great control of strengthening activities within the client's tolerance level.[2,5]

Turbulence

Turbulence is an irregular movement of the water. Turbulence is produced by a moving body. Turbulence can be used as a form of resistance to exercise in the pool. The quicker the movement, the greater the turbulence, which means an exercise can be increased by increasing the speed of exercise. Swimming in water is easier than walking in water because the body is more streamlined when swimming, whereas an upright body walking creates more turbulence.[2,5]

Surface Tension

The surface tension of water behaves in a different manner than the body of water. The surface of water acts like a membrane under tension. This can be demonstrated by floating a needle on the surface of the water. The density of a needle is greater than that of water. Therefore, it should sink. But, the tension at the surface is great enough to support the needle. Once the surface tension has been broken, the needle will sink. Surface tension acts as a resistance to movement when a limb is partially submerged and the surface tension has to be broken by the movement.[2,5]

Summary

The many physical principles that govern the behavior of water are complex. The beneficial physiologic effects of water start immediately with immersion. Heat transfer begins. The hydrostatic pressure effects also begin immediately. The work of breathing is increased with immersion. The pressure of water forces the central return of lymph fluid and pushes out extracellular fluid. The force of water alters blood volume and blood pressure. Tissue circulation is increased and temperature regulation comes into play. While immersed in warm water, blood is shunted to the surface of the skin, thereby increasing circulation to large muscles. This change in the circulatory patterns assists in the healing of musculoskeletal injuries. The whole human body is profoundly affected with immersion into water.

Aquatic Rehabilitation Techniques and Education

Therapeutic aquatic techniques have been evolving over the last century. Today, aquatic rehabilitation techniques are being developed and adapted from land-based techniques such as aquatic Feldenkrais®, PNF, and shiatsu. The older, more traditional aquatic rehabilitation techniques like the Bad Ragaz Ring method and the Halliwick method, originated in Europe in the 1950s and continue to be used in this country. Individuals have created their own brand of aquatic techniques, which they named after themselves, such as the Dolan method, the Burdenko method, and the Jahara technique.

Aquatic rehabilitation education most typically comes after graduation in the form of conferences and workshops. Discipline-specific organizations, such as the American Therapeutic Recreation Association (ATRA) and the American Physical Therapy Association, host aquatic specialty workshops. Fitness organizations that sponsor aquatic workshops include the Aquatic Exercise Association, United States Water Fitness Association, Young Men's Christian Association (YMCA), and American College of Sports Medicine.

Aquatic safety education may be obtained by the American Red Cross, Ellis and Associates, and the YMCA. Aquatic facilities may sponsor their own staff safety training courses for emergency procedures.

The Aquatic Therapy and Rehabilitation Institute hosts a multi-disciplinary aquatic rehabilitation conference. A variety of aquatic techniques and diagnostic-specific treatment are showcased by a diverse group of presenters. Some of the techniques may include Bad Ragaz, Feldenkrais®, aquatic PNF, Halliwick method, Watsu®, Jaharra, Wassertanzen™, and the Burdenko method. Diagnosis-specific courses may relate to back injuries, multiple sclerosis, arthritis, shoulder injuries, knee injuries, and neurologic disorders.

Vertical Exercise

Preliminary research has suggested that people can become physically fit faster by exercising in water vertically rather that horizontally.[2,5] When the body is vertical, the heart has to pump against gravity, which causes it to pump with greater force, thereby strengthening the heart muscle. When the heart is stronger, it does not have to work as hard to circulate the same or a greater volume of blood. As a result, the vertical water exerciser has more energy and improved stamina after less training time than a swimmer who is horizontal.

Vertical exercise also allows a person to burn calories more efficiently. Since a swimmer is face down in the water, his or her airflow is restricted by 20%. This decreases the oxygen to the muscle tissue, causing the muscles to be less efficient, because they are getting only partial oxygen. Since the upright water exerciser receives the maximum benefits of oxygen to the muscles, like the land jogger, he or she can become physically fit faster than a swimmer. Additionally, larger muscles, including buttocks and thighs, burn more calories. The vertical water exerciser is in a position to use a full range of motion with the upper trunk and the lower body while utilizing optimal oxygen, thereby burning more calories in less time. Calorie burning translates into weight (fat) loss, a final benefit of vertical exercising in warm water. Since warm water temperature is the same as the skin's, individuals who exercise in water need not retain a layer of subcutaneous fat to stay warm, as do cold water competitive swimmers. Consequently, exercising in warm water places a person at risk for hyperthermia.

Bad Ragaz

The Bad Ragaz technique, ultimately influenced by proprioceptive neuromuscular facilitation (PNF), was developed in Bad Ragaz, Switzerland, in the 1930s. In 1957, Dr. Knupfers of Wilbad, Germany, refined the method to utilize flotation devices to provide support to the patient's head, neck, hips, and extremities while floating in a horizontal position either supine or prone. The patient exercised in simple one-dimensional planes. By 1967, Bridget Davis and Verena Laggatt incorporated PNF patterns, resulting in the Bad Ragaz technique known today. The therapist acts as a fixed pivot point, moving the patient in spiral or PNF diagonal patterns. This technique, in its purest form, is resistive and used to increase strength and improve joint stabilization, coordination, and gross and fine motor control. Neurologic, orthopedic, and surgical patients benefit from Bad Ragaz.

Training in the Bad Ragaz technique occurs in a variety of settings, including national and individual organizations, which offer training workshops ranging from one to four days. No certification is offered. However, continuing education credits are given, including a certificate of participation. Aquatic service providers generally learn Bad Ragaz techniques to exercise the arms, legs, and trunk for joint stabilization and muscle strengthening.

Halliwick Method

The Halliwick method offers two clearly defined elements: swimming instruction and therapy.[5] This method was developed in England by James Macmillan, an engineer, who developed the Halliwick method using his knowledge of competitive swimming skills and engineering principles. Additionally, he observed handicapped persons in the water and had many discussions with Berta Bobath, a physical therapist, and her husband Karel Bobath, a neuropsychiatrist, who both developed the Bobath neurodevelopmental treatment approach.[8] The Bobaths influenced MacMillan in the development of the Halliwick method by teaching him their neurodevelopmental treatment approach. The Halliwick method has been used to instruct children to swim, while improving balance and trunk control.

The Halliwick Ten Point Program, which involves the swimming element, is divided into four phases: adjustment, balance restoration, inhibition, and facilitation. Adjustment concerns adaptation to being in the water. The adjustment phase has two points. Mental adjustment, the first point, deals with a client becoming comfortable in the water. Disengagement, the second point, focuses on the client becoming independent from the instructor. Once the client is adjusted to the water, he or she is advanced to the next phase, balance restoration. Balance restoration involves four points of the Ten Point Program: vertical rotation control, lateral rotation control, combined rotation control, and mental inversion. Vertical rotation control, the third point, is the client's ability to control movement from a vertical or standing position in the water to a horizontal position of supine floating, then returning to a standing position. Lateral rotation control, the fourth point, is the client's ability to control rolling in the water. This step is considered the most important maneuver for the client to learn, since it is a safety maneuver that could save the person's life. Combined rotation control, the fifth point, is the client's ability to achieve any position in the water. The client can combine and control vertical and lateral rotation. Mental inversion, the sixth point, "is the process of learning that the force of buoyancy is an upward thrust that brings objects, including the client, to the surface of the water."[5] On completion of balance restoration, the client progresses to the third phase, inhibition. This phase, which is the seventh point, challenges the client's ability to regain lost equilibrium caused by turbulence or movement in the water. With mastery of inhibition, clients are advanced to the final phase, facilitation. Mastery of the facilitation phase implies that a client is able to control movement through water. Turbulent glide, the eighth point, is concerned with holding a balanced position while passively gliding through water. Simple progression, the ninth point, looks at holding a basic balanced position while gliding through water and beginning gentle movements to assist simple propulsion. Basic movement, the tenth point, is the final process of teaching the client actual swimming strokes.

The therapy element of Halliwick utilizes static positioning, dynamic positioning, eye deviations, and turbulence as well as phases from the Ten Point Program to challenge the client's physical abilities.

The two levels of training are available in the United States: the basic course and the advanced course. These courses are sponsored by a variety of groups, such as universities and professional organizations. The basic course offers instruction in the Ten Point Program for instructing swimming to normal individuals and the disabled. The advanced course offers instruction specific to the rehabilitation of ill or injured clients.

Task-Type Training Approach

The task-type training approach (TTTA) was developed for clients who had a stroke. This approach also is effective with those who have had brain injuries. The purpose of TTTA is to improve the client's functional skills. This is accomplished by working in functional positions with functional activities. Clients are encouraged to actively participate in solving their own problems of movement. Seven general principles for the task-type training approach guide therapists as they develop treatment programs for their clients:

1. Work in the shallowest water that can be tolerated.
2. Practice functional activities as a whole.
3. Systematically remove the external stabilization provided clients.

4. Encourage stabilizing contractions in upright positions with the movement of selected body segments.
5. Encourage quick, reciprocal movement.
6. Encourage active movement problem solving.
7. Gradually increase the difficulty of the task.

Because of the properties of water, activities can be graded from simple to more complex. Activities can be made more challenging, thus increasing a client's ability to perform functional tasks, or they can be simplified for the client with severe problems.[5]

Watsu®

Watsu® is a technique developed in 1980 in northern California by Harold Dull, a Zen shiatsu instructor. Originally created as a water massage or wellness technique, the term *Watsu* comes from water and shiatsu. Watsu® consists of slow, rhythmic movements to stretch, increase range of motion, normalize tone, and improve relaxation of the recipient. The client passively floats on his or her back while the Watsu® practitioner moves the client around a warm pool (90°F or more). The lulling movements of Watsu® are relaxing. For example, a client with fibromyalgia who has a tendency to be in a constant state of excitement or in a sympathetic autonomic nervous response could receive a Watsu® with the desired outcome of relaxation, as seen during parasympathetic response.

The Worldwide Aquatic Bodywork Association (WABA), located in Middletown, California, professional organizations, and others sponsor local, regional, and international workshops for training in Watsu®. To become a practitioner, one must complete 330 hours of Watsu® training with documentation of Watsu® practical experience. Regular continuing education is necessary for maintaining the Watsu® certification.

Land Techniques Turned Aquatic

Numerous individuals have adapted typically land-based techniques for use in water, including aquatic Feldenkrais®, aquatic PNF, and the biomechanic approach. Feldenkrais® is a technique that requires a client to move in ways not typically performed in a normal day. The moves are slow and calculated. Aquatic PNF is a hands-on, hands-off resistive technique, where a client performs resisted diagonal patterns. Either the therapist or the water provides the resistance. The biomechanic approach is exercising in simple planes.

Namesake Aquatic Techniques

Several aquatic techniques have been named for the individuals who developed them. The Burdenko method was developed by Russian exercise physiologist Igor Burdenko. Mario Jahara Pinto, a Brazilian Zen shiatsu teacher and Watsu® practitioner, developed the Jahara method. The Dolan method was developed by Mary Dolan, a certified therapeutic recreation specialist.

The Burdenko Method

The Burdenko method is a hands-off technique that may or may not use equipment to promote rehabilitation, training, or conditioning. The Burdenko method takes place in a variety of positions and depths of water. The Burdenko method initially was utilized in the treatment of high-level athletes. Burdenko's techniques now are utilized in many settings for a diverse clientele incorporating land and water exercises into a comprehensive program.

The Jahara Method

The Jahara method is a hands-on passive technique performed while a client floats on his or her back. Styrofoam floatation devices are placed under the knees to offer support to the body and a sense of freedom to both the practitioner and client. The use of floatation devices makes it easy to maneuver any body type into gentle, flowing stretches and movements. Jahara provides relaxation similar to Watsu®, although it sometimes is considered more gentle.

The Dolan Method

The Dolan method is a deep-water method of teaching autistic children to swim. Autistic children's perseverative behavior is discouraged as they learn about their bodies while immersed in water. Swimming skills gradually are introduced until child is able to swim.[9]

References

1. Skinner AT, Thomson AM. *Duffield's Exercise in Water.* London: Bailliere Tindall; 1983:4–196.

2. Becker BE, Cole AJ. *Comprehensive Aquatic Therapy.* Boston: Butter-worth–Heinemann; 1997:1–179.
3. American Red Cross. *Community Water Safety.* Washington, DC: The American National Red Cross; 1995:1–5.
4. Harrison RA, Hillman M, Bulstrode S. Loading of the lower limb when walking partially immersed. *Physiotherapy.* 1992; 78:165.
5. Ruoti RG, Morris DM, Cole AJ. *Aquatic Rehabilitation.* Philadel-phia: Lippincott; 1997:3–402.
6. Bates A, Hanson N. *Aquatic Exercise Therapy.* Philadelphia: W.B. Saunders; 1996:1–311.
7. Campion MR. *Hydrotherapy Principles and Practice.* Boston: Butter-worth–Heinemann; 1997:3–326.
8. Hopkins HL, Smith HD. *Willard and Spackman's Occupational Therapy,* 6th ed. Philadelphia: Lippincott; 1983:114–116.
9. Spowal B. *The Dolan Method: Teaching the Child with Autism to Swim* [thesis]. Cincinnati, OH: University of Cincinnati, College of Education; 1991.

CHAPTER 5

Aquatic Exercise Instructor

Helen M. Tilden

Introduction

Water accommodates many abilities and performance levels for rehabilitation and aquatic exercise, and it is a venue for referral from therapists following discharge from therapy.[1] Rehabilitation (see Appendix B, Glossary) to restore function often begins within 24 hours of an injury or immediately after a wound is healed.[1,2] Aquatic exercise is versatile and may be used as a wellness program for a person who cannot tolerate aerobic activities on land or as an integral part of an athlete's cross training schedule for fitness. The versatility of water to accommodate rehabilitation and exercise has contributed to the growth and interest in the field of aquatics.

Growth and interest often necessitate change, education, and training. This is demonstrated by the profusion of multilevel educational conferences, training programs, and workshops for physical therapists, occupational therapists, and others on the multidisciplinary team. These educational and training sessions teach new and standard aquatic therapy techniques. Through multilevel education, the aquatic field continues to grow, with basic education for the therapist just beginning an aquatic therapy career and continuing education to advance the knowledge base of the experienced therapist.

The aquatic exercise field is in state of change. Referrals to aquatic exercise classes following discharge from therapy have altered the participant profile in community aquatic classes and increased the responsibilities for the aquatic exercise instructor (AEI). Prior to the health care changes of the past decade (i.e., managed care), most aquatic participants presented as deconditioned adults or older adults with goals to be healthy and physically fit. The class participant today may be a person who is less fit and less independent with goals to maintain skills acquired in therapy and improve or maintain fitness.[3] The participant is empowered or forced to assume responsibility to maintain independence and a home exercise program (HEP).

Many factors contribute to a less independent person attending an aquatic exercise class. Some are the decreased length of stay in the hospital, reduced number of therapy visits, and family members participating in the recovery process at home. Aquatic exercise classes are a cost-effective, convenient method to improve strength, balance, aerobic capacity, and overall well-being.[4] Aquatic exercise classes are not the same or a substitute for prescribed therapy.

If therapy is ordered for an outpatient, the family and client face a multidimensional decision. To maintain or continue newly earned skills or pain management techniques, they may consider cost, transportation, location, and the time of day therapy is scheduled. These factors may be a temptation to cancel the visits to the therapist and seek a less expensive or more convenient program provided by an aquatic instructor or other nonlicensed personnel. As the use of nonlicensed personnel escalates, it is important for the aquatic instructor to educate the client and family that aquatic exercise classes are not therapy.

Post-Rehabilitation Referrals

Referral to aquatic exercise classes for maintenance of skills acquired from therapy may pose problems for the client and the instructor. One is the misconception that the class is therapy or an extension of therapy. The aquatic instructor is no substitute for nor equivalent to a licensed therapist who assesses, evaluates, and changes the plan of care to ensure maximum functional restoration and independence. To prevent fraud, the aquatic instructor must represent the class or program as group classes for the purpose of recreation, fitness, or wellness and not one-to-one therapy. Other possible problems that may arise from referrals are the mobility, fatigue, balance, and overall fitness level of the client. This adds to the existing broad level of participants in the group exercise class and the instructor's responsibility to acquire information and training specific to each participant's condition.

Aquatic exercise classes are available on-site at a hospital or clinic or at off-site locations such as a health club or YMCA. On-site referrals to the aquatic exercise instructor from the rehabilitation team provide cash flow to help cover fixed costs. Benefits are positive for the facility and the client, because classes sponsored by the facility are a known entity with trained instructors in a reputable, proven program format, such as the Arthritis Foundation aquatic program. Off-site referrals also meet the needs of the client with the added benefit of a location near the home or workplace. In either setting, the AEI maintains contact with the rehabilitation team if there is a change in status or questions arise.

Aquatic exercise classes are recreational in design and purpose and consist of a format that includes active exercise for health and overall well-being, program adherence, injury prevention, and independence. Most clients who attend aquatic exercise classes want to prevent injury or stay healthy. Aquatic classes usually are taught by a nonlicensed person, known as an *aquatic exercise instructor* or *aquatic personal trainer*. The goals of the participant determine the appropriate aquatic class, which may include aqua aerobics, gentle flexibility classes, water walking, or deep-water exercise.

Participants usually join a class near their home or work place, but they may choose to work with an aquatic personal trainer. The sessions are arranged privately and fees are paid by the client. This is one-on-one instruction, private training versus a group class. The personal trainer performs no manual techniques nor designs a program for the acute phase of injury recovery or rehabilitation nor applies thermal modalities. The aquatic personal trainer generally works with clients who have no serious medical problems or musculoskeletal disorders. This type of instruction, although one-to-one, is not therapy.

If the client is recovering from surgery or illness, a referral to aquatic classes generally comes from the therapist, rheumatologist, surgeon, neurologist, or other health care provider. Flexibility, function, and fitness are typical goals for clients referred to aquatic classes. Examples of referrals are persons with arthritis, fibromyalgia, multiple sclerosis, or other chronic diseases; joint replacement; sports injury; cardiac disease; or head injury. It is possible for the aquatic instructor to receive a referral from any member of the continuum (see Figure 5–1).

Therapists often attend aquatic training provided by organizations such as the Arthritis Foundation, National Multiple Sclerosis Society, or YMCA, but it is rarely cost effective for a therapist to teach wellness classes. The specialty training by these organizations is targeted to nonlicensed personnel. The training includes an overview of pathology, but the focus is an appropriate exercise regimen for the specific condition to promote program adherence, independence, and enjoyment. The aquatic class is taught in a group setting.

Group classes are designed to maintain or improve fitness, provide socialization, and accommodate a wide scope of participants.[5] Although the class may include people with chronic diseases, back pain, recent injury, or recent surgery, words such as *therapeutic, patient,* or *therapy* are not used in marketing or during class. Benefits occur based on the participant's ability, compliance, attitude, contribution, interpretation, and understanding of the program's value.

Aquatic classes benefit the participant and the health care industry. Together with affordable cost, availability in multiple locations, and a social atmosphere, programs continue to grow in the United States because they meet the needs for most participants referred to a exercise regimen after therapy. The aquatic program of the Arthritis Foundation is an example. With 84,430 participants in 1995, it now has classes in all 50 states and more than 185,000 participants.[4]

The aquatic programs of the Arthritis Foundation/YMCA and the National Multiple Sclerosis Society have specific participant classification guidelines in the manual provided at the training, based on status of joint degeneration or type of arthritis or, for multiple sclerosis, disease progression or type. Participants in aquatic exercise classes are also described as beginner, intermediate, or advanced. Classification includes level of fitness or wellness and ability to perform the exercises. Those requiring one-on-one therapy are not included in these groups.

Clients in aquatic exercise classes are mobile with or without assistive devices and require a minimum of assistance, if any, to enter and exit the pool. They are cleared by a doctor or therapist if there is a preexisting condition such as arthritis.[6] If there is no illness or

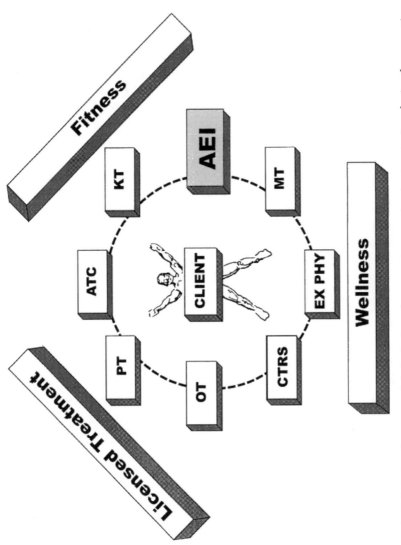

FIGURE 5–1. Lyton model depicting the aquatic exercise instructor's role in the aquatic continuum of care.

condition, no referral is needed, they simply join a class. Beginners are moderately deconditioned and most likely have not exercised regularly for an extended period of time. Intermediates have been in an exercise class on a regular basis and are minimally deconditioned. Those in advanced classes have developed endurance and may be "more fit" than others. More strenuous activities and longer work sessions are incorporated into the advanced-level classes.

The properties of water permit movement that is easier than on land. The client exercises at an intensity based on ability and endurance. Balance, gait, strength, coordination, posture, breath control, increased endurance, and ease of movement are a few of the benefits of aquatic classes that promote independence, fitness, or wellness. The aquatic instructor provides the plan, adaptation, and demonstration of exercises to accommodate the range of abilities in the class. Community classes are a cost-effective, affordable method that offers the client an active role in the plan of exercise, progression, and leisure activities. The fees are paid by the client and not an insurance reimbursement program.

Aquatic classes span a range of classes that include water walking to enhance balance and coordination, deep-water running and aqua aerobics classes to promote cardiovascular endurance. All classes are designed with the client performing active exercise with no manipulation or prescription for activity from the aquatic instructor. Classes include general areas of development, such as improve joint action, increase efficiency of movement, improve circulation, build muscle strength, or reduce stress and fatigue. Aquatic exercise classes contribute to the reduction of risk factors associated with a sedentary lifestyle such as hypertension, heart disease, and diabetes.

Community aquatic classes include exercises performed by the client with progression and equipment use as tolerated. The focus of the instructor's lesson plan is on the abilities of the client to perform the exercises, program adherence, and the client's goals for overall wellness or fitness.[7,8] Outcomes and safety are also considered for program growth and enjoyment. A typical lesson plan follows.

Exercises

1. Active or active-assistive (performed totally by the participant).
2. Pain free.

3. Performed smoothly and controlled by participant.
4. Focused on functional and physical fitness.
5. Within participant's ability to perform.
6. Structured to include contraindications and modifications for physical limitations and disease-specific counterproductive movement.

Progression for Walking

1. Increase intensity as tolerated; for example, walk in longer strides, walk faster, or walk in patterns such as letter *S*, letter *W*, box, or circle.
2. Water jog.
3. Exercise combinations.
4. Buoyancy or surface area equipment, if tolerated.

Focus

1. Joint range of motion.
2. Muscle endurance and strength for balanced upper and lower body workout.
3. Cardiovascular endurance, if indicated.
4. Muscle power and speed.
5. Reaction time, coordination, balance.
6. Static and dynamic movements.
7. Proprioception.
8. Posture and body mechanics.
9. Education, such as joint protection, energy conservation, pain.
10. Enjoyment.

Optimal Outcomes

1. Program adherence.
2. Customer satisfaction (i.e., meeting personal goals).
3. Reduction in diseases of a sedentary lifestyle.
4. Reduction in secondary and tertiary symptoms of chronic conditions.

Deep-water activities are for those who are able to swim. Utilize shallow water if participant is unable to swim.

Training and Certification

The new participant profile adds the responsibility for the instructor to attend workshops for additional training and to accurately represent his or her education, skills, and qualifications to protect the client and prevent fraud. The AEI also may elect to take a certification examination to document basic skills. Workshops, training, and certification are a bridge to the rehabilitation team for post-rehabilitation referrals. Water safety training, special population training (e.g., the Arthritis Foundation aquatic program) combined with an interest in the health and wellness of the public increase the potential for post-rehab referrals from the health care team.

Safety and responsibility begin with water safety training. The aquatic environment poses dangers not present on land. Drowning, falls on a slippery deck, fatigue, increase in blood pressure, or a reaction to medication due to water temperature pose dangers not posed by land-based exercise programs. Training in first aid and CPR are important for the instructor to be an active member of the emergency response team to save a life or prevent further injury. If the AEI works with children, the program should include infant and child CPR in addition to adult CPR. Swimming skills to respond in an aquatic emergency are vital to protect the participant. Water safety courses are available through Red Cross, National Parks and Recreation, or YMCA, as are programs for CPR, water safety, and first aid.

Aquatic workshops, training programs, and certification are available for the instructor to teach community classes without therapist supervision. These courses and training enhance the possibility of referrals from the therapist when the instructor is well prepared. Courses are provided through aqua aerobic workshops and certification by organizations such as the Aquatic Exercise Association, the Arthritis Foundation. and the YMCA.

Many training and certifying organizations exist. Some test knowledge acquired through self-study or courses taught by the certifying body targeted to the examination. This type of training or certification usually provides a stimulus for the organizations' continuing education programs. A strong, consistent foundation may or may not follow the certification process. Inquire about the type of literature and educational materials provided and used for lecture as well as the faculty teaching the course and conducting the examination.

Assess what you will learn (skills and training), the reputation of the organization, and how this course or certification will enhance your programs and income before you pay the fee. Consider the amount and cost of continuing education required to maintain the certificate. This additional investment of time and money is often granted only by the certifying body.

Programs and training sponsored by the Arthritis Foundation/ YMCA Aquatic Program (AFYAP), the National Multiple Sclerosis Society (aquatic training), and the YMCA do not require therapist supervision. All are nationally and internationally recognized organizations with training or certification for aqua aerobics and special populations such as those with arthritis, fibromyalgia, or multiple sclerosis. The programs have reasonable fees to register, usually less than $100 for an eight-hour course. The programs are designed by health care professionals and aquatic instructors to reflect information based on research and expert opinion, not personal experience, a company, or product program. The programs meet a safety, educational, and fitness level for most participants enrolled in aquatic classes. The integrity of such certification and training protect the instructor, the participant, and the facility.

Liability

Health care changes have created a challenge for the rehabilitation team with the use of nonlicensed personnel. Predictions in *Rehab Management*[3] have made an impact on the design of community aquatic programs and the therapists' practice. Increased use of extenders of care, integration of "functional therapy," and an investment toward injury or illness prevention programs are three examples. As a health care extender, the aquatic exercise instructor is a link to wellness and injury prevention programs after discharge from therapy.

Therapy visits are limited in today's managed care environment. When the patient is not functioning maximally but exercise still is indicated, some hospitals and clinics utilize health care extenders, aides, technicians, or those with other titles. Titles are merely titles and may be bestowed through attendance at a workshop or other means for nonlicensed personnel. *Specialist* and *assistant* are two titles that may confuse patients and should not be used to imply the employee is a licensed therapist.

The use of nonlicensed personnel creates an obligation for the facility to inform clients if employees are not licensed therapists. The facility must also provide a job description and delineate the role to prevent fraud (see Appendix C). When nonlicensed personnel are employed as health care extenders, the facility must consider not only the welfare of the patient but the liability.

Liability is part of everyday life. For example, a person who drives a car without a license assumes the liability that, if stopped by the authorities, a fine may be imposed; but a lawsuit is unlikely. Utilizing a person without a license to work as a "therapist" is a liability and the facility hiring nonlicensed personnel must consider the safety of the patient. Knowledge and skill levels vary. That is, the aquatic instructor and the facility are liable, with litigation a possible consequence if injury occurs. Malpractice and litigation take its toll, financially and personally, if one works without a license in a specific scope of practice. The impact and cost to health care is significant, but the impact is enormous on the lives of the person working without the license and the person injured or deceived as a result of it.

The aquatic instructor may be employed as an extender but not as a substitute for a therapist. The education and training of the instructor are not the consistent, educational curriculum and preparation of a therapist. This creates a responsibility for the employer to evaluate credentials, training, and certificates presented by nonlicensed personnel for employment. Hands-on experience, in-house on-the-job training, and off-site or conference training are important but no substitute for a curriculum that issues a license to practice and the responsibilities associated with it. Certificates that state "has attended," "has completed," "has demonstrated," and other nebulous terms are not diplomas to certify educational preparation for licensure.

Weekend courses and passing a test from an organization or certifying body is no substitute for a license in health care. For example, an elementary education teacher may have an advanced degree in education but is not licensed in the health care field and, therefore, cannot practice under the guise of "the same as" or "equal to" a doctor, therapist, or other health care professional during the acute phase of rehabilitation. This is fraudulent, unlawful, and may place the client at risk. At the time of treatment, the person is a patient, vulnerable and in a compromised state, not one discharged from therapy to an aquatic exercise class for a fitness regimen.

However, nonlicensed does not mean unaccountable. Valid training and certification from organizations with a reputation for accurate information assist in the preparation to teach aquatic exercise classes. It is the responsibility of the employer to evaluate whether or not titles, product certifications, and trainings are accepted by the facility and do not misrepresent the status of the aquatic exercise instructor. Local or regional trainings may be valid only where obtained and product certifications may offer restrictions to practice only with the confines of the product liability.

Halliwick, Bad Ragaz, Watsu®, and aquatic Feldenkrais® are four training workshops taken by nonlicensed personnel with an expectation to practice beyond or outside the fitness role. Although licensed therapists attend these workshops and utilize these techniques, the nonlicensed person who performs the techniques during or after class is performing one-on-one treatment. This is a liability when the nonlicensed person does not understand the rationale, impact, and outcome to the participant.

Acceptance and Recognition

Therapists work one on one or in small groups and receive third-party reimbursement. Generally instructors are paid an hourly wage per class or a salary for aquatic exercise in a group setting. Therapists are trained and educated to assess, prescribe, alter, and evaluate the client.[1,9] Aquatic instructors make broad general assessments. Without an appropriate educational background, weekend courses and certificates of attendance acquired by aquatic instructors do not produce competency or acceptance equal to the licensed therapist.

Much of this lack of acceptance and career development is justified, due to the variety of educational backgrounds and preparation of the aquatic instructors and those conducting the workshops they attend. Instructors learn and ultimately teach what they agree with, enjoy, and understand. If the workshop is beyond their level of education to understand the information, they merely learn applications and techniques and do not fully understand why they are doing what they are doing.

The relevance and validity of "therapy" workshops targeted to instructors also are suspect when these are conducted by individuals who lack the clinical and educational expertise to fully understand the information they present. With these variables, the educational background of the instructor and the person conducting the workshop plus any underlying objective, it is unreasonable to assume the aquatic instructor is equal to a therapist or will be accepted and recognized as such in the realm of rehabilitation or aquatic therapy.

Career Development

Career development and success in the health care field is measured by specific entry or advanced degrees, status, employer, and industry recognition. The measure of success for an aquatic instructor often is contracts for videos and books, industry (peer) recognition, program growth, and presenting weekend workshops. Although aquatic instructors have no license or degree in therapy, they are vital to the Lyton model for the aquatic continuum of care. The health care team refers the client to aquatic classes following therapy for a lifetime of independence and health. Additionally, the books and videos they produce assist others in the field of aquatics with choreography, class themes, variety for interest and program adherence, and overall information about the field of aquatics.

Independent Practice

There is a distinct difference between education and training. This is the decisive factor that determines who may practice as a therapist and who is an instructor. Training is skills based and usually focuses on one subject or topic; education is knowledge based and designed to stimulate thinking and creativity as one builds the knowledge base through experience and application of skill. The objective of training is to bring a diverse group to the same level of skill for the immediate application of a specific task or function, whereas the objective of education is an understanding and the application of skills. Licensure following the completion of a prescribed course of education is required for practice in the health care field, which includes therapy; for example, physicians, physical therapists, and occupational therapists are licensed. Therapists complete a specific educational curriculum to prepare for licensure in order to work independently in private practice or as an employee. Additionally, they may obtain advanced degrees to enter fields such as research or education. The primary barriers for aquatic instructors to practice independently and receive reimbursement from third-party payers are the lack of licensure and the varied educational backgrounds compared to the standardized education of a therapist. Licensure determines a scope of practice and is regulated by a body such as a state and the state's practice act.

Although most instructors acquire training or certification from one of the many training or certifying organizations in the United States, no training or education is required to work as an aquatic instructor. No license is available for aquatic instructors. The training, certification, and education of a aquatic personal trainer is as varied as that of the aquatic exercise instructor and there is no license for a personal trainer. Without licensure, standardized education, and a recognized body to regulate the industry, it is impossible to determine a written scope of practice for instructors and other nonlicensed personnel working in the aquatic environment.

Training for instructors usually involves one- or two-day workshops and presents a limited amount of information that includes general physiology and an overview of a specific disease pathology, process, or disability; fundamental knowledge about indicated and contraindicated exercises; and parameters, goals, and objectives of the program. A licensed health care professional, such as a physical or occupational therapist, is included in the training process to ensure accurate information and promote a relationship with the health care team. An aquatic instructor may be a member of the training team to provide practical, innovative, and diverse information to design enjoyable group classes. Regardless of the number of continuing education units or certificates of attendance, this type of training does not equal the education of the therapist. The knowledge and skills learned by the instructors enable them to conduct aquatic exercise classes that promote health and wellness for a quality of life.

Summary

Aquatic exercise is broad in scope and accommodates the needs of many with a focus on fitness or wellness. Aquatic physical therapy is explicit and specified for the many phases of an illness or condition with a specific plan for rehabilitation.[1,9]

Rehabilitation is a collaborative effort with the patient at the center of a multidisciplinary team of specialists that includes the family members, friends, and community resources. The physical medicine team consists of athletic trainers, physical and occupational therapists, recreational therapists, kinesotherapists, as well as nurses, assistants, and other specialists. They treat athletes, persons with chronic illness, person with total hip replacements, and a myriad of other clients wanting to regain maximum independence.

At the head of the team are the client and the doctor, who may be a neurologist, orthopedist, or physiatrist. The roles may be complex, but each member of the team contributes to the outcome, which often includes aquatics for a transition from non-weight-bearing to weight-bearing activities and a referral to an aquatic fitness or wellness program.

It is critical to the success of any team to encourage and create an environment of respect for the contribution of all members, who in turn refer clients to aquatic exercise classes for a fitness program to enjoy life and prevent sedentary illnesses, injury, or infirmity.

Interaction with Roxanna

Prior to an operation, Roxanna's options are an aqua aerobics class or the Arthritis Foundation/YMCA aquatic program, if her arthritis is too painful to tolerate the duration and intensity of an aqua aerobics class. Fitness and health goals are reviewed at three-month intervals to adjust the workout to her needs and ability. She will move to a class of increased duration and intensity if and when indicated. Or, she will transfer to a lower level class if indicated with exercises modified with changes in speed and lever length.

In an aqua aerobics class, the goals are flexibility, cardiorespiratory endurance, and increase of muscle strength and endurance. The goals of the AFYAP are flexibility and independence. In aqua aerobics and AFYAP, all exercises are performed by the participant as active or active with assistance. If Roxanna can swim, some deep-water exercises are appropriate to relieve the weight from her joints, reduce pain, add variety, and change the intensity from the shallow water lesson plan.

Immediately following her operation, Roxanna would receive physical therapy and possibly occupational therapy. Following discharge from therapy, she would enter the AFYAP program with a referral from her surgeon or therapist. The goals are flexibility, pain-free movement, and independence. If movement remains pain free and endurance increases, progression to an aqua aerobics class is appropriate. In either class for Roxanna, the health- and skill-related elements of fitness are the focus for independence and wellness.

The Role of the Aquatic Exercise Instructor in the Continuum of Care

The objective of the aquatic exercise instructor is to enhance and support the physiological and psychological aspects of rehabilitation following discharge from therapy as a result of illness, injury, surgery, or disease.

The AEI's function is to teach aquatic exercise classes to increase or produce efficiency of movement, the activities of daily living, and a healthy mind and body. The goals of these classes are to

1. Reduce the risk of cardiac and other diseases that result from a sedentary lifestyle.
2. Reduce risk of complications of chronic illness or disability, such as contractures, decubiti, muscle atrophy, and infections.
3. Reduce stress, isolation, depression.
4. Increase self-esteem, a feeling of well-being.
5. Increase socialization.
6. Increase the participant's perceived quality of life.
7. Increase the participant's program adherence.
8. Increase the participant's quality of sleep.
9. Increase the participant's level of fitness or wellness.

The participants in such classes could be

1. Older adults.
2. Those with low back pain.
3. Deconditioned adults.
4. Those with chronic illness, such as arthritis, Parkinson's disease, multiple sclerosis, fibromyalgia, post-polio syndrome, or chronic fatigue syndrome.
5. Those recovering from recent surgery or injury.

6. Pregnant women and those who have recently given birth.
7. Others by referral or recommendation from the multidisciplinary team for a fitness regimen.
8. Children, such as in youth fitness classes.

The instruction uses verbal, written, or hand cues and encourages, praises, and supports the participants' goals.

The AEI designs and teaches programs to

1. Promote wellness or fitness.
2. Preserve or improve independence and function.
3. Reduce the incidence or severity of complications of long-term disease, illness, or injury.
4. Promote muscle strength and overall body conditioning.
5. Educate and inform the participant.
6. Strategically work with the multidisciplinary team.

Comparing the Environment of an Aquatic Fitness Instructor to an Aquatic Physical Therapist

1. All exercises are performed by client (no hands-on), whereas the aquatic physical therapist (PT) may add weights, perform massage, manipulate limbs, regulate or change exercises, provide resistance, or use passive exercises.
2. Temperature range is tepid, 80–88°, whereas the aquatic PT may use temperatures exceeding 88°, as indicated. See temperature chart in Appendix B.
3. Focus is on physical fitness or independence and mobility, whereas aquatic physical therapy focuses on quantifiable functional restoration.
4. Fitness assessment is broad and general, whereas aquatic physical therapy involves evaluation by testing and measurement; application and use of modalities; assessment of program design, progression, and results; written documentation; referral; and discharge.
5. Broad general goals, whereas aquatic physical therapy is specific to need and ability.
6. Does not draw conclusions from data, whereas the aquatic PT uses data for functional, financial, and other outcomes for independence and restoration.

7. Receives participant into group sessions for fitness and socialization, whereas PTs provide care one to one in acute, habilitative, rehabilitative, and preventive stages.

References

1. Cunningham J. Historical review of aquatics and physical therapy. In Cirullo JA (ed.). *Orthopaedic Physical Therapy Clinics of North America*. Philadelphia: W.B. Saunders; June 1994:83–94.
2. Koury JM. *Aquatic Therapy Programming*. Champaign, IL: Human Kinetics, 1996.
3. Sallicido R. Competence in the new millennium. *Rehab Management*. August–September 1996:23–24.
4. Arthritis Foundation/YMCA Aquatic Program (AFYAP) and AFYAP PLUS *Instructor Manual*, Atlanta, GA: Arthritis Foundation; 1996.
5. U.S. Department of Health and Human Services. *Physical Activity and Health: A Report of the Surgeon General*. Atlanta, GA: U.S. Department of Health and Human Services, Centers for Disease Control and Prevention, National Center for Chronic Disease Prevention and Health Promotion; 1996.
6. Arthritis Foundation/YMCA Aquatic Program *Guidelines and Procedures Manual*. Atlanta, GA: Arthritis Foundation; 1996.
7. Greenberg JS, Pargman D. *Physical Fitness: A Wellness Approach*. Englewood Cliffs, NJ: Prentice-Hall; 1989.
8. Hoeger W, Hoeger SA. *Lifetime Physical Fitness and Wellness*, 4th ed. Englewood, CO: Morton Publishing; 1995:11–31.
9. American Physical Therapy Association. *Statement on Health Care Reform: Who Are Physical Therapists?* Alexandria, VA: APTA; 1995.

CHAPTER 6

Certified Athletic Trainer

Charlotte O. Norton

Introduction

The roots of the athletic training profession can be traced to Grecian times. Historically, with the rise of organized sports, Greek civilization promoted the Olympic games. Coaches, trainers, and physicians came to the forefront to assist the athlete in the pursuit of optimum performance.[1] Herodicus of Megara, a physician and athletic trainer, was regarded as one of the finest Greek trainers. His claim to fame came as the teacher of Hippocrates, "father of modern medicine."[2] Nearly 300 years later, Galen, a Roman physician, wrote extensively about the beneficial effects of proper diet, rest, exercise, and abstinence from drink and sexual indulgence as prequisites for physical conditioning.[3,4]

Athletic training as we know it today evolved from the late 19th century. The first athletic trainers used elementary techniques with little knowledge of anatomy and the pathology of athletic injury. Historically, the term *training* implies the coaching or teaching; therefore, considerable confusion has existed with the terms *training, athletic training, trainer,* and *athletic trainer.*[3] In 1997, the National Athletic Trainers' Association (NATA) defined an *athletic trainer* as "an allied health professional who has a bachelor's degree from an accredited

college/university, has fulfilled the requirements for certification as established by the NATA Board of Certification (BOC), and passed the NATABOC certification examination administered by the NATABOC. The certified athletic trainer works under the direction of a licensed physician when practicing the art and science of athletic training."[5]

The establishment of intercollegiate and interscholastic athletics in the United States brought rapid change in the athletic training profession. The National Athletic Trainers Association was formed in 1950 to establish professional standards for the athletic trainer. Today, the certified athletic trainer (ATC) plays a vital role in the prevention, recognition, treatment, and rehabilitation of injuries to the physically active.

Education and Qualifications

Athletic training education has followed two paths: curriculum and internship. Curriculum programs are usually housed within Exercise and Sport Science or Health and Physical Education Departments and follow specific academic guidelines for accreditation. The Commission on Accreditation of Allied Health Education Programs (CAAHEP) is responsible for awarding the accreditation. Curriculum students are required to be supervised by an ATC for 800 contact hours. Internship programs provide athletic training experience by requiring fewer core courses but 1500 supervised hours.

The NATA recently established new criteria that will eliminate the internship option for certification in the year 2004. The NATA Education Council's Competencies in Education and Clinical Education Committees developed standards of athletic training educational competencies for the health care of the physically active. These "competencies" will provide guidelines and standards for curriculum development and the education of entry-level athletic training students. They address the cognitive, psychomotor, and affective objectives, including knowledge and intellectual skills, manipulative and motor skills, and attitudes and values, respectively. Required course work includes

1. Acute care of injury and illness.
2. Assessment and evaluation.
3. General medical conditions and disabilities.
4. Health care administration.

5. Nutritional aspects of injury and illness.
6. Pathology of injuries and illnesses.
7. Pharmacology.
8. Professional development and responsibilities.
9. Psychosocial intervention and referral.
10. Risk management and injury prevention.
11. Therapeutic exercise.
12. Therapeutic modalities.

On successful completion of the required education and practical experience the student athletic trainer is eligible for the national certification exam. Every state, except Texas, recognizes this certification. Texas established its own certification procedure. The NATA Governmental Relations Department reports that 39 states regulate athletic training in some manner. Currently, 21 states have licensure, 8 have certification, 6 have registration, and 4 have exemption. Once certified by the NATABOC, the ATC is required to obtain eight continuing education units every three years to remain certified.

Traditionally, ATCs have practiced within the interscholastic, intercollegiate, or professional sports arena. Most professional sports teams, colleges, and universities have an athletic training staff, the members of which work in conjunction with the team physician to provide health care for the athletes. In the 1980s, many ATCs began working in outpatient rehabilitation clinics. In this setting, ATCs often work under the supervision of a physical therapist in the provision of physical therapy services. State practice acts generally guide the use of an ATC in the outpatient clinic. Many clinical ATCs also are instrumental in the development of outreach programs to provide athletic training services to high schools or community sporting events. These community events may involve participants ranging in age from youth to seniors. Some ATCs have created a niche working with the injured worker, creating the term *industrial athlete*. Many of the principles applied to the rehabilitation of the athlete can be used to return the injured worker back to work.

Aquatic Rehabilitation Training

The recent competency guidelines established by the NATA for athletic training education include aquatic athletic training as a contemporary therapeutic exercise. We surveyed 10 schools. Two schools

provide basic aquatic rehabilitation information as a component of the athletic training curriculum and one school uses aquatic therapy routinely in the rehabilitation of athletic injuries.

Based on this informal survey, we suggest that most ATCs gain their aquatic experience via on the job training or continuing education. An ATC can select from a variety of continuing education courses designed for multidisciplinary audiences. Courses also are taught at national, regional, or state athletic training conferences. The ATC can learn techniques such as Watsu®, Feldenkrais®, Bad Ragaz, Burdenko method, and Ai Chi. Additionally, the Arthritis Foundation and National Multiple Sclerosis Society offer certification courses that ATCs attend to teach aquatic exercise classes for populations with these diseases.

With the increase of athletes using water for rehabilitation and cross training, safety is a concern for the athlete as well as the ATC. Many universities and high schools have natatoriums. Some training rooms are now equipped with single-user pool systems to provide convenience for the athlete. It is important for the athletic training staff to develop emergency procedures specific to their facility.

The Role of the ATC in the Continuum of Care

In the 1980s, ATCs increased the use of water for rehabilitation and cross training to maintain optimal performance and prevent overuse injuries. In the traditional college, university, or high school settings, the ATC generally works with a physician to promote health and prevent injuries. The ATC assesses, coordinates, and directs the health care and rehabilitation of the athlete. This may include aquatic rehabilitation. The ATC employed in the outpatient sports medicine clinic may provide aquatic rehabilitation services in conjunction with land-based rehabilitation. The contemporary ATC also plays a vital role in the wellness and prevention of injury in the physically active. This may include aquatic fitness or cross training and wellness classes.

The primary role of the aquatic ATC is to provide the physically active individual with an opportunity to use the properties of water for rehabilitation with the goal of returning to their previous activity. For example, the basketball player who undergoes a surgical

repair of his or her anterior cruciate ligament can begin aquatic athletic training immediately with an occlusive dressing to protect the incision site. Gait training in the pool can be initiated within the first week after surgery, depending on the athlete's weight bearing status. Similarly, plyometrics and sport specific activities can be initiated in the pool at earlier phases of the rehabilitation program than on land. Initiation of early activity helps prevent depression and encourages earlier return to sport-specific activities.

ATCs may also develop aquatic cross training programs for the physically active. An example is preseason conditioning for a volleyball team. The ATC and coach work together to develop a sports-specific program in shallow or deep water for preseason conditioning, including cardiovascular endurance, sports-specific strengthening, and plyometrics. This type of program helps prevent overuse injuries. It also provides an opportunity to prevent burnout and boredom in athletes.

In some states, practice acts allow the ATC to perform aquatic rehabilitation services for the physically active under the direction of a physical therapist for reimbursement by third-party payers. This practice will differ from facility to facility depending on protocols and state practice acts for both professionals.

Barriers to Provision of Aquatic Athletic Training Services

Professional issues challenging the role of the ATC are not new. Generally, these are present in the outpatient clinic setting and related to reimbursement issues. Lack of standardized aquatic therapy education within athletic training curriculums causes many ATCs to use the water without understanding the hydrodynamic principles. Also, the lack of clear role delineation among the multiple disciplines that provide aquatic services creates confusion among consumers, aquatic professionals, and third-party payers.

Athletic Trainers and the Lyton Model

The ATC works closely with physicians, physical therapists, and occupational therapists (see Figure 6-1). Many ATCs work independently to

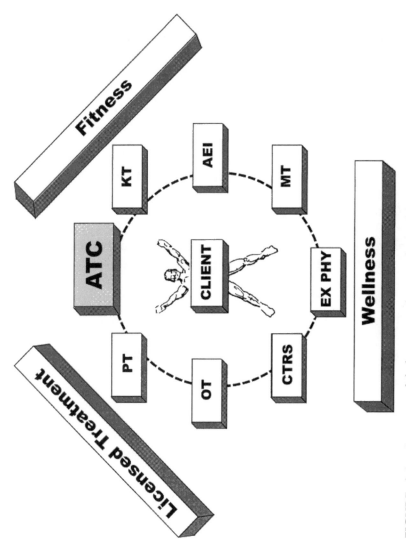

FIGURE 6–1.   Lyton model depicting the certified athletic trainer's role in the aquatic continuum of care.

provide rehabilitation services for the athletes at their institution. An ATC who does not possess expertise in the aquatic arena may refer an athlete to an aquatic physical therapist. The ATC also may interact with the aquatic fitness professional in the development of cross training programs for the physically active. Written and verbal communication between the disciplines is important as often these services are provided out of the athletic training room.

Interaction with Roxanna

Roxanna may encounter an ATC in an outpatient clinic setting. An ATC may teach a post-rehab class for total joint replacements or the Arthritis Foundation aquatic program.

References

1. Harris HA. *Greek Athletes and Athletics*. London: Hutchinson and Company; 1964.
2. Durant W. *Caesar and Christ*. New York: Simon and Schuster; 1944.
3. Arnheim DD. *Modern Principles of Athletic Training*. St. Louis: Times Mirror/Mosby; 1989.
4. O'Shea ME. *A History of the National Athletic Trainers' Association*. Greenville, NC: NATA; 1980.
5. National Athletic Trainers Association Board of Certification. *Credentialing Information: Entry Level Requirements*. Dallas, TX: NATA; 1997.

CHAPTER 7

Exercise Physiologist

Carol A. Kennedy

This chapter discusses the role of an exercise physiologist (EP) in caring for clients within the aquatic rehabilitation setting. An overview of licensure, certification, scope of practice, and how EPs are prepared academically to be involved in aquatic therapy will be reviewed. Finally, a specific case study will illustrate the contribution of the EP as a member of the team of health care professionals.

Licensure

Recognition of competency in the medical field usually is based on a medical or allied health license. Physicians, nurses, physical therapists, occupational therapists, and the like are examples of medical employees who have a license to perform their work. Most of their professions have set standards of practice that outline their specific privileges and limitations.

The fitness profession, on the other hand, has no set level of competency. The term *exercise physiologist*, once applied to the Ph.D. scientist and researcher but now is a common description for certain graduate-trained personnel who work in clinical settings such as hospitals, clinics, and some fitness facilities. According to Rosche,[1] insurance companies in the United States will pay for treatment of diseases diagnosed by health care professionals licensed to practice within their particular state. As of today, only one state in the United States licenses clinical EPs. The pros and cons of licensure for EPs has been discussed at several American College of Sports Medicine (ACSM) national meetings. Currently, several states are considering licensure but only for the clinical EP.[2]

A licensed health care professional has passed a licensure exam. Many EPs possess certifications to practice. However, certification is very different from licensure. Licensure is generally state regulated and includes disciplinary action. Certification documents one's status and qualification without offering disciplinary action in the event of malpractice. Certification is not acceptable to third-party payers for many types of services performed within the health care industry. Therefore, an EP must have a referral from a qualified, licensed professional for third-party reimbursement.

The majority of exercise professionals who work in the clinical setting are trained at the graduate level (MS, MA, Ph.D.) with experience specific to exercise physiology. In July 1995, the Louisiana state legislature passed a bill (Senate Bill 597) regulating clinical EPs. The bill primarily sets the scope of practice for cardiac rehab services, but issues such as weight management, diabetes, and cancer are mentioned within the text. One would assume that licensure automatically would ensure reimbursement, but this has not occurred in Louisiana. Several clinics have reported that they have not increased third-party billing due to this change. Licensure does not guarantee reimbursement. However, Louisiana may ensure a clinical EP's place in the medical field at a future date. ACSM hopes the CEP will be accepted for third-party reimbursement.

Certification

With Louisiana being the only state to license fitness professionals, it is important to understand certifications of different organizations in order to learn what the EP brings to the aquatic continuum of care. These skills will vary with the type of certification and training the exercise professional acquires. Certification provides health and fitness professionals with public recognition of their knowledge, technical skills, and experience in their particular field or specialty. It certifies that the individual is qualified to practice in accordance with the standards deemed to be essential by the certified body.[3,4]

Since there is no national certification for aquatic exercise physiology, it will be important to compare the other fitness organization certifications and pay particular attention to the practical experience of the EP in the area of aquatic exercise physiology. Three criteria often are used to judge whether one is qualified to assist someone on basic health, wellness, and exercise-related issues:

1. Formal academic preparation.
2. Professional experience.
3. Professional certification.

It has been estimated that more than 60 organizations offer some form of certification for health and fitness professionals.[5] Four of the more prominent certifying organizations are listed below. ACSM and ACE are the only two organizations that have written tests that have been checked for reliability and validity. The organizations are presented here with a brief overview of what they offer in terms of water exercise.

Aerobics and Fitness Association of America

The Aerobics and Fitness Association of America (AFAA) offers two types of certification: group exercise and personal training. The AFAA offers an Aqua Fitness Educational Workshop, where it presents its standards and guidelines for basic water exercise and aqua fitness but does not offer certification of those teaching water exercise.

American College of Sports Medicine

The American College of Sports Medicine (ACSM) offers three levels of certification within two specific tracks: a clinical track and a health and fitness track. No specific certification on water exercise is offered but knowledge of exercise in the water is included in the knowledge, skills, and attributes requirements.

American Council on Exercise

The American Council on Exercise (ACE) offers four types of certification: group exercise, personal training, lifestyle and weight management, and for a clinical exercise specialist. The ACE offers continuing education credits for water fitness that allows the student to get a water exercise specialty certificate after completing 15 hours of training in water fitness.

Young Men's Christian Association

The YMCA offers 10 levels of health and fitness certification: fitness leader, fitness instructor, strength training instructor, strength training director, youth fitness instructor, healthy back instructor, prenatal and postpartum exercise instructor, fitness walking instructor, weight management consultant, and water fitness instructor.

Each of these organizations has an important place in the fitness field. However, the EP should have at least one certification through ACSM, which is seen as the "gold standard" in the field of sports medicine and fitness. Several water fitness certifications are available on the market; however, the standards associated with land-based exercise certification are more rigorous and offer increased credibility. Proof of attending workshops or seminars on water fitness and certifications from one of the preceding organizations provide an alternative for demonstrating an aquatic knowledge base. The water certifications are inconsistent in the knowledge base needed in the area of exercise science and assessment, which is critical for the blend of fitness and medicine.

The big difference between an EP and a fitness instructor is that the EP has had formal training or education at the university level in exercise prescription and fitness assessments. In 1970, the ACSM was the first organization to identify a goal of increasing the competency of individuals involved in health and fitness and cardiovascular rehabilitative exercise programs. With increased public awareness of the benefits of exercise, the ACSM also saw the importance of consumers being able to recognize professional competence.

With publication of the first edition of the *ACSM's Guidelines for Graded Exercise Testing and Prescription*, the college was able to set the standards and objectives for its clinical track certifications. Since 1975, more than 6000 individuals have been certified in one or more of the clinical tracks, which consist of three levels. At the height of the health and fitness awakening in the early 1980s, the ACSM introduced its health and fitness track certifications for those working with apparently healthy and disease-controlled individuals. In only 15 years, more than 11,000 health or fitness professionals have been certified by the ACSM. The qualifications for ACSM certification contain a practical portion that requires assessment or demonstration and a written test calling for more in-depth knowledge than the other certifications. There are established prerequisites for ACSM certification, whereas the other certifications require only CPR certification prior to taking the test. According to ACSM,[6] certification at a given level requires the candidate to have a knowledge and skill base commensurate with that level of performance. In addition, higher levels of certification incorporate the knowledge and skills associated with previous designated levels.

Although no strict prerequisite experience or level of education is required for taking all ACSM certification examinations, each level of certification has been developed to include specific knowledge and skills at designated levels of employment. Within the ACSM clinical track the exercise specialist certification is the most popular and has the following prerequisites:

- Minimum of 4 months or 600 hours of practical experience in a clinical exercise program.
- Baccalaureate degree in an allied health field or equivalent.
- Ability to execute an accurate individualized prescription of activities for patients referred to clinical exercise programs.
- Ability to effectively educate or council patients regarding activity and lifestyle issues.

Within the health/fitness track, the health fitness instructor certification is the most popular and has the following prerequisites:

- Educational training comparable to an undergraduate or graduate degree in a health and fitness curriculum or closely related field.
- Adequate knowledge and skill in risk factor and health status identification, fitness appraisal, and exercise prescription.
- Practical hands-on experience with exercise leadership.
- Experience in lifestyle behavior modification skills.

In terms of relating this to aquatic exercise, it would be important to ensure that some of the hands-on practical experience was in the area of aquatics. The certification will help assure knowledge in exercise science but not within the field of aquatic exercise physiology. This knowledge can be achieved by doing an internship or working with a program where there is a focus on aquatic exercise physiology. Minimal information on exercising in the water is tested in the ACSM certification process in both the written and practical exams. However, passing an ACSM test shows a higher level of knowledge in the content of exercise prescription.

Scope of Practice

Outlined here is the general scope of practice of an EP who has completed a degree in the field of exercise and sports science.

Assessments

A large portion of the exercise curriculum is dedicated to performing basic assessments and assisting participants with setting goals. Included in these assessments are body composition analysis using skinfolds, underwater weighing and various other anthroprometric tests, flexibility testing using a sit and reach box or goniometer measurements, muscular strength and endurance tests, and cardiorespiratory testing. Very clear guidelines have been established by the ACSM for testing individuals before they begin an exercise. The guidelines also list when a physician needs to be present (see Table 7–1).

A general interpretation of the recommendations is that EPs can test apparently healthy people who want to engage in moderate activity. However, if they are older or want to engage in vigorous activity, then a stress test with a physician present is recommended. The majority of EPs are trained to test vital signs including blood pressure measurements. Additionally, they assess and analyze the health history information and determine who is apparently healthy, at risk, or has known disease (see Table 7–2). Clinical EPs certified by the ACSM as exercise specialists also can attach EKG electrodes and assist with stress testing. Interpretation of testing results through putting these to use in the exercise setting is a part of their training. For example, when they learn a patient's VO_2 max, they can convert this to METS and tell the patient how to work at 50–75% VO_2 max while exercising on a treadmill. In other words, the EP assists to quantify the amount of exercise the client is performing and assist with proper exercise progression.

TABLE 7-1
ACSM Recommendations for Medical Examination and Exercise Testing Prior to Participation.

A. Medical examination and clinical exercise test recommended prior to:

	Apparently Healthy		Increased Risk[a]		Known Disease[b]
	Younger[c]	Older	No Symptoms	Symptoms	
Moderate exercise[d]	No[e]	No	No	Yes[f]	Yes
Vigorous exercise[g]	No	Yes[f]	Yes	Yes	Yes

[a]Persons with one or more risk factors (see Table 7–2) or one or more signs or symptoms.

[b]Persons with known cardiac, pulmonary, or metabolic disease.

[c]Younger implies <40 years for men, <50 years for women.

[d]Moderate exercise is defined by an intensity of 40–60% VO_2 max; if intensity is uncertain, moderate exercise may alternately be defined as an intensity well within the individual's current capacity, one that can be sustained for a prolonged period of time, that is, 60 minutes, that has a gradual initiation and progression, and generally is noncompetitive.

[e]A "no" response means that an item is deemed "not necessary." The "no" response does not mean that the item should not be done.

[f]A "yes" response means that an item is recommended. For physician supervision, this suggests that a physician should be in close proximity and readily available if there would be an emergent need.

[g]Vigorous exercise is defined by an exercise intensity >60% VO_2 max; if intensity is uncertain, vigorous exercise may be alternately defined as exercise intense enough to represent a substantial cardiorespiratory challenge or if it results in fatigue within 20 minutes.

Source: Reprinted with permission from American College of Sports Medicine. *ACSM Guidelines for Graded Exercise Testing and Prescription*, 5th ed. Baltimore: Williams and Wilkins; 1995.

Clinical Exercise Therapy

An actual prescription of exercise to patients who are under the care of a physician, whether it be preventive or rehabilitative, metabolic or orthopedic, depending on the referring situation, is another role of the EP. Exercise usually consists of one or more of, but not limited to, the following: aerobic conditioning, flexibility, resistance exercise, active range of motion, and movement education. Examples include walking, biking, treadmill walking or running, supervised exercise, one-on-one training, group exercise, resistance training, and video instruction.

capabilities. The aquatic EP who has experience doing this kind of training in the water would be especially helpful to the aquatic therapy providers.

Administration and Management

Those who work in health care settings often find themselves working in both clinical and administrative capacities, whether it is as a department head or the owner-director of a rehabilitation facility. Many health clubs are forming alliances with health insurance providers that pay their policyholders to join and participate in member clubs.[8] The EP can serve as the liaison for these organizations' staffs or lead the sessions at the club that involve the patients. Often, facilities (such as pools) are the limiting factor for health providers. An alliance with community resources for fitness and wellness is occurring in many parts of the country. Wellness programs are not just a fad but here to stay. The International Health, Racquet and Sportsclub Association (IHRSA) published a booklet on the economic benefits of regular exercise. It states: "the Surgeon General, along with the Department of Health and Human Services, has stated that 70% of all illnesses are due to lifestyle-related causes; in fact, one-half of all medical costs are attributable to illnesses that could be prevented. Clearly, there's a need for corporations to help their employees establish a healthy lifestyle."[9] The EP often is the link between insurance companies and clubs in terms of management and administration of fitness programs that cross over from the clinical to preventive area.

General Exercise Programs

Apparently healthy adults and children may require or request exercise services outside the realm of the clinical referral. This area deals with preventive services by exercise specialists, such as lifestyle intervention, activity planning, nutritional assessment and planning, and conditioning techniques such as endurance or resistive exercise training. Ideally, the EP ought to be able to refer these patients to certified fitness instructors, exercise leaders, or personal trainers they are familiar with in the community. The role of the EP is to seek out these community resources. Many fitness facilities have no trained instructors (especially in water fitness). It is important for the clinical providers to reach out and educate the general public, just as the fitness professional, to mainstream clients in a healthy manner.[10]

Academic Preparation for an Exercise Physiologist

The academic preparation to practice as an EP depends on the university program and its requirements for graduation. There is no standard curriculum for the EP. The following is an overview of what most EPs study. It is important to note the differences, but core courses for exercise physiology majors in the undergraduate programs include

- Anatomy.
- Exercise physiology.
- Basic testing and assessment.
- Application of exercise principles.
- Organic chemistry.
- Physics.
- Biomechanics.
- Research techniques.

A graduate program will expand on physiology and add classes in cardiovascular physiology, respiratory physiology, and the same physiology of human movement class that most medical students take. A course in EKG and stress testing is included in this advanced preparation. Practical application of these skills is part of the exercise science curriculum. Many universities have adult fitness service programs that help train students and offer a service to the community. At Colorado State University (CSU), for example, the adult fitness program is considered phase three of the local hospitals cardiac rehabilitation program. Patients are referred to the CSU Adult Fitness Program when the physician feels they are ready to enter phase three. Unlike the typical health club, in these programs, blood pressures often is checked before and after exercise and a crash cart is available for a possible cardiac event. Many facilities refer to their programs as *cardiac rehabilitation programs*. Usually, an EP on the clinical track will obtain exercise specialist certification or Certified Exercise Physiologist (CEP) through ACSM.

The concept of personal training recently was added to curriculums. Personal training involves using goal setting, exercise prescription and progression, and one-to-one training with clients as they work toward their goals. Personal training is becoming quite popular but training and certification varies. It is difficult for the client to assess who has proper training because the term *personal trainer* is not licensed or trademarked. There is no standard definition or qualifications. The client must assess the aquatic personal trainer's academic and practical experience. Many personal trainers will possess the ACSM health fitness instructor certification, as this certifies they can perform fitness testing and assessment within the guidelines written by ACSM.

To join the medical field as professionals, EPs must be able to "quantify" the success of the exercise and one-on-one training and document the results. For example, an exercise prescription by an EP might read as follows:

Cardiorespiratory fitness goals: Increase VO_2 max from 28 ml/kg/min to 32 ml/kg/min.

Body composition goals: Decrease overall body fat from 29% fat to 25% fat with an increase in lean body weight and a decrease in fat weight.

Flexibility: Decrease goniometer measurement of hamstring flexibility from 28°–20°.

Muscular strength and endurance: Push up test goals from 10–15 per minute with good form, and curl up goals from 20–30 per minute.

The ability to quantify and prescribe exercise is what separates the EP from the fitness instructor or group exercise leader. If specific measurable parameters are not being set, then a licensed professional will have difficulty referring a patient to the EP and justifying that referral to a third-party payer. Therefore, making sure an EP can set specific, measurable goals is essential for success as a part of the aquatic continuum of care (Figure 7–1). This probably is the most important part of their training that prepares EPs to work in the medical field.

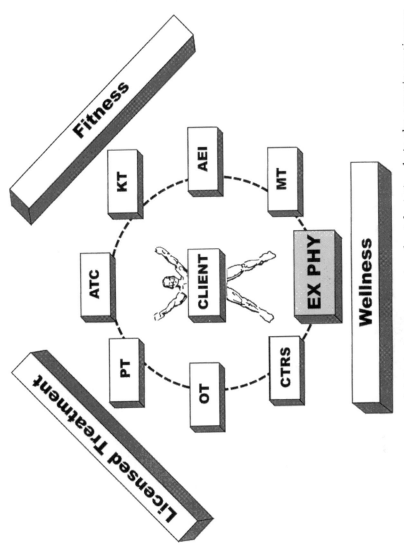

FIGURE 7–1. Lyton model depicting the exercise physiologist's role in the aquatic continuum of care.

Interaction with Roxanna

Roxanna is a 64-year-old woman who suffers from a combination of osteoarthritis and rheumatoid arthritis. She weighs 205 pounds and is 5 feet tall. The initial diagnosis of arthritis was made at age 43. She was told she would need to lose weight and exercise three to five days per week. At age 56, Roxanna fell, broke her right hip, and received a total hip replacement. Roxanna can bathe and dress herself while sitting. Housekeeping is somewhat difficult; however, it all gets done. Roxanna drives a car and is able to shop. The neighborhood teenagers are paid to keep up the yardwork. Walking is painful and she has a noticeable limp. Roxanna uses a cane for long distance ambulating and walking out of the house.

How might an EP assist Roxanna and the rest of the medical team working with her? Most likely, a body composition analysis would be performed on Roxanna and specific measurable goals would be set. For example, if Roxanna has 39% body fat, a realistic goal of losing ½% per month would be established and a specific weight calculated to represent what that would be on the scale. Roxanna may not lose any weight right away but her composition should be changing. After a month, she may weigh the same but have 2 pounds more lean body weight and 2 pounds less body fat, which is significant. Setting more specific parameters for weight control would be one way the EP could contribute to Roxanna's case.

Since Roxanna has some physical limitations due to her osteoarthritis, it may be difficult for her to reach a level of intensity that would benefit her cardiorespiratory system and increase her overall fitness. The EP could help Roxanna set up heart rate and rate of perceived exertion parameters during her workout. For example, her target heart rate could be calculated and the rate of perceived exertion reviewed so Roxanna would have effective workouts to help her reach her goals. The EP can calculate energy expenditure based on metabolic equivalent (MET) levels.

The EP also could inform Roxanna on which exercises could enhance her daily living activities. Since housekeeping is somewhat difficult, it would be important to help her stay independent by working on the specific movements that Roxanna uses on a daily basis and creating exercises that simulate these movements. Of course, the EP will need health information from the physician on her overall state of health beyond her physical limitations. Further information from the physical and occupational therapists about recommended movement patterns and exercises, as well as contraindicated exercises and movement patterns, will be needed. Once this has been established, the EP can work to bring Roxanna into a regular setting within the community or her home by teaching her the skills she needs to work in these settings. Often medical providers tell patients to "get more exercise" without giving them the skills for success with exercise. This truly is the role of the EP. Once clients know "how" to exercise and understand how to modify such exercise to account for their specific limitations, they can enter mainstream aquatic programs or fitness facilities or work on their own at home.

References

1. Roche C. *The Insurance Reimbursement Manual for America's Body Workers, Body Therapists, and Massage Professionals*, 2nd ed. Cupertino, CA: Bodytherapy Business Institute; 1991.
2. Durak E, Shapiro A. *The Ins and Outs of Medical Insurance Billing*, 2nd ed. Santa Barbara, CA: Medical Health and Fitness Publication; 1996.
3. Neiman D. *Exercise Testing and Prescription, A Health Related Approach.* Mountain View, CA: Mayfield; 1999:66–69.
4. Peterson JA, Bryant CX, Stevenson R. Making professional certification work for your facility. *Fitness Management.* July 1996:36–38.
5. DuBois PC. Certification: How to spot the real thing. *Fitness Management.* August 1995:46–48.
6. American College of Sports Medicine. *ACSM's Guidelines for Graded Exercise Testing and Prescription*, 5th ed. Baltimore: William and Wilkins; 1995.
7. Cinque C. Back pain prescription: Out of bed and into the gym. *Physician and Sports Medicine.* 1989;17(9):185–188.
8. Gandolfo C. Health insurance subsidizes fitness. *Fitness Management.* June 1998:52–54.
9. Waters C. *The Economic Benefits of Regular Exercise.* New York: International Health; Racquet and Sportsclub Association; 1997:3.
10. Kennedy C, Flegel M. In the swim: How water fitness professionals can work with the medical community. *IDEA Today.* May 1994: 56–57.

duty. Funding was provided by the federal government. By 1947, corrective therapy had become an important part of the physical rehabilitation component within the VA medical system. In 1953, the American Corrective Therapy Association (the predecessor of the AKTA) recognized the need for a credentialing process and adopted a certification examination to establish a consistent level of competency.[4] The establishment of credentials and applicable academic programs documents the evolution of this career field. In 1980, the clinical training requirements increased from 400 to 1000 hours. In 1982, the industry established the Council on Professional Standards for Kinesiotherapy (CPSK). Continuing education became mandatory in 1986 for KTs to maintain their current registration. In 1987, the Professional Evaluation Service (PES), a national testing organization, was contracted to standardize and administer the national certification examination for KTs. The AKTA regulates national registration, provides and oversees continuing education, and governs university programs. In 1988, corrective therapy was renamed *kinesiotherapy* to better define its role as a provider of therapeutic exercise, and the profession's governing body became known as the American Kinesiotherapy Association.[4]

The primary goal of aquatic kinesiotherapy is to improve function by increasing one or more parameters of fitness: strength, flexibility, cardiovascular endurance, and muscular endurance.[1,2] A KT provides instruction under the direction of a physician. The aquatic KT begins therapy early in the rehabilitation phase when active movement is indicated, especially when movement on land is difficult—either painful or of poor quality in strength and biomechanics. An indicator for aquatic kinesiotherapy is a weight-bearing sensitivity or an inability to move an extremity fully against gravity. The KT will use exercises in the water to increase range of movement of an extremity, strengthen muscles, and improve balance, coordination, and the level of conditioning. Aquatic kinesiotherapy is used as a precursor to or to enhance a land-based therapeutic exercise program. Aquatic kinesiotherapy also is used to reduce chronic pain and increase aerobic and muscular endurance for increased function.

Bed rest is not prescribed today, as it once was in the treatment for conditions such as low back pain. Today, we are more aware of the detrimental effects of disease and inactivity. Corcorcan states that a muscle exerting less than 20% of its maximum force begins to atrophy, whereas exercise at 20–30% of maximum force will preserve a muscle's strength.[5] Corcoran also reports that virtually every organized body system promptly and progressively deteriorates in inactivity.[5]

Often people who have pain fear movement and this fear makes their pain worse. Because chest-deep water alleviates about 70% of the effects of gravity, movement is easier and often less painful. For example, individuals who have chronic pain and are sedentary are at risk for developing diseases such as heart disease, obesity, and osteoporosis. Aquatic kinesiotherapy with a transition into an independent water exercise program can afford the individual with chronic pain the opportunity for exercise, especially aerobic exercise, that would be too painful or difficult on land.[6]

In the areas of industrial fitness and work reconditioning, KTs have used aquatic kinesiotherapy as reconditioning exercise dating back to the 1970s. Usually an individual with a work-related injury is referred for aquatic kinesiotherapy with a KT when the reconditioning aspect of rehabilitation is indicated. The use of aquatic kinesiotherapy in general varies with the exposure physicians have had with this discipline.

Kinesiotherapy consists of whole-body exercise combined with therapeutic exercise for a specific injured area, as well as exercise and prevention education. Aquatic kinesiotherapy most often is implemented initially and then integrated with a land therapeutic exercise program. Emphasis is placed on restoration of functional skills such as walking, lifting, carrying, sitting, or standing, preparing the worker to return to his or her job.

Within the profession of kinesiotherapy, there is variation of treatment among KTs specializing in aquatics kinesiotherapy. The variation is determined by the population and type of facility served by a particular institution. Also, a KT's skills and interests may dictate the direction taken in acquiring specialized training in aquatic kinesiotherapy. KTs work in concert with other therapists and health care professionals in many settings. In aquatic kinesiotherapy, within the VA medical system, the pool most often is serviced by the kinesiotherapy department, while other disciplines, such as physical therapy and recreation therapy, have access to the pool as needed. KTs within the VA medical center program work with a variety of diagnostic groups such as people with low back pain, arthritis, cardiac disease, chronic pain, and other medical conditions affecting an individual's level of conditioning and function.[7]

Completing of an accredited baccalaureate program and success-fully passing the certification examination allows one to become a registered kinesiotherapist (RKT). RKTs who meet the CPSK continuing education requirements qualify for listing in the national registry. To maintain registration, KTs must earn 50 continuing education units every three years. These continuing education units must be approved by AKTA's director of continuing education.[8,9]

Education and Credentials

The educational preparation of the KT involves graduation from an accredited university or college. The accreditation is maintained by the Committee on Accreditation of Educational Programs for Kinesiotherapy. In 1998, there were six accredited programs in the United States and according to the American Kinesiotherapy Association mission statement, an estimated 2000 individuals are registered and employed as KTs.[1] The kinesiotherapy course of study typically is an integrated curriculum with kinesiotherapy theory, physical education, exercise science, and practical hands-on experience. Other kinesiotherapy course work may include human anatomy and physiology, neuroanatomy and physiology, perceptual motor development, exercise physiology, human muscle physiology, kinesiology or applied anatomy or biomechanics, general psychology, test and measurements, research methods, statistics, motor learning, adaptive physical education, therapeutics, and organization and administration. Following successful completion of the core course work, students must complete a 1000-hour clinical training internship under the direct supervision of a registered KT. The internship may be in rehabilitation clinics; hospitals; mental health, nursing, and wellness centers; or schools that provide special services.

Aquatic Kinesiotherapy Training

Training in aquatic kinesiotherapy varies among the accredited programs. Some schools, such as the University of Toledo, have kinesiotherapy clinics on campus that utilize the university swimming pool for therapy. At universities that have aquatic kinesiotherapy programs on campus, the kinesiotherapy student gains early exposure and training in aquatic kinesiotherapy. In those schools that do not offer university-based aquatic training, students must seek continuing education courses specific to aquatic kinesiotherapy independent of the university setting. Aquatic continuing education courses for KTs are generally multidisciplinary and not specific to kinesiotherapy.

The Role of Kinesiotherapy in the Continuum of Care

The role of a KT is to provide extended physical conditioning and education to clients who require treatment beyond physical therapy. Generally, clients are medically stable and able to tolerate increased levels of activity following the initial injury or illness. KTs provide services under the prescription of a licensed physician and, therefore, are accountable to that physician regarding their actions and those of their subordinates. KTs are certified by the American Kinesiotherapy Association and are required to engage in continuing education to maintain certification.

After receiving a prescription from a physician, a KT evaluates a client by taking detailed information, including age and medical history of the injury or illness that resulted in the physician's referral. A physical evaluation is completed regarding muscle strength, flexibility, cardiovascular fitness, and functional mobility. A psychosocial evaluation also is completed related to the appropriateness of behavior, ability to integrate with a group, capability of task planning and goal-directed behavior, orientation to environment, capacity and appropriateness of affect, motivation, and assessment of patient family interaction.

The KT interprets the data to develop a treatment plan of physical exercise and education. Physical exercise may improve strength, flexibility, mobility, cardiovascular fitness, and coordination. Education consists of a home exercise program for the client and instructions regarding proper body mechanics. For example, after a client with an injured back who becomes medically stable can participate in an aquatic back exercise program in an individualized group setting, under the direction of the KT. Body mechanics education would include how to properly push, pull, lift, and carry objects safely without causing further injury. The aquatic exercises would increase abdominal strength and improve trunk stabilization to minimize back pain.

KTs also teach water exercise classes for clients with particular problems such as arthritis groups, chronic pain groups, or substance abuse groups. In these classes, the KT acts as instructor of a class designed to increase general wellness and not as a therapist.

By and large, a KT renders services in an individualized group setting, as in the following example. Three individuals have had total hip replacements, and each has individualized needs: The first client is overweight, the second demonstrates poor body mechanics, and the third has poor balance. The KT will group these three individuals together, as a total hip replacement group, but will tailor treatment to their individualized needs. In some settings, one patient will have a hip replacement, one lower back pain, and one a shoulder injury. Each individual will perform an aquatic kinesiotherapy routine specific to their condition.

The VA medical system, to date, is the largest employer of KTs. KTs also may be employed in other settings, including rehabilitation clinics, sports medicine clinics, industrial fitness and work hardening programs, nursing homes, and adaptive physical education programs. New Hampshire's state labor board recognizes kinesiotherapy as a viable and reimbursable service for injured workers receiving worker's compensation. New Hampshire, Ohio, Oregon, and Virginia host specific insurance plans and health maintenance organizations that recognize and reimburse kinesiotherapy services. As of 1999, KTs do not receive Medicare reimbursement.

Barriers to the Provision of Aquatic KT Services

Insurance companies that require licensed therapists for therapy services do not reimburse facilities for nonlicensed kinesiotherapy. Only three states—New Hampshire, Ohio, and Virginia—recognize the profession of kinesiotherapy. Therefore, KTs often practice as nonlicensed physical therapy aides under the direction of a physical therapist, in which case the services are considered and billed as physical therapy. In 1997, the VA system became bound to state practice act laws. If a given state does not recognize a KT as a licensed medical provider, the KT must work under the supervision of a licensed therapist. For example, in New Mexico, a KT may work for the VA but must work under the supervision of a physical therapist. The role of a KT in this setting is that of physical therapy aide. In New Hampshire, KTs are not licensed, but have been recognized by entities such as the State Labor Board, which enables the billing of kinesiotherapy directly under workers' compensation and by vocational rehabilitation.

Additional barriers limit the provision of aquatic kinesiotherapy services, such as no standardized aquatic education for KTs and the lack of clear role definition between KTs and other professionals who provide aquatic kinesiotherapy services. KTs as a group are small in number and, at the present time, are recognized by few states.

When working in clinical settings in states that do not recognize their services, KTs work as aides or technicians under the direction and supervision of licensed therapists. KTs may work independent of other licensed clinical professionals as exercise specialists, fitness instructors, or aquatic specialists when working in wellness or fitness settings. When performing these duties, they are recognized as KTs.

KTs and the Lyton Model

The contribution to rehabilitation by KTs in the Lyton model (Figure 8–1) and as a whole is relatively small due to the disproportionate number of KTs compared to physical therapists, occupational therapists, or recreational therapists. The role of kinesiotherapy is to provide reconditioning and treat with exercise and education. The philosophy of kinesiotherapy can be summed up by the motto "improvement through movement."

KTs work in concert with other therapists and health care professionals in many settings. The role of the KT is to provide reconditioning activities or extend what licensed physical and occupational therapists have begun. In the VA medical system, KTs provide aquatic kinesiotherapy services in contrast to other disciplines and receive referrals directly from the physician. In the private sector, a KT likely will receive referrals from other health care professionals when reconditioning is indicated.

Interaction with Roxanna

Roxanna has undergone total hip replacement surgery and has completed physical therapy. In her physical therapy, she learned to transfer safely, increase hip girdle strength, and improve her gait. Occupational

for muscle endurance and aerobic conditioning is initiated and deep-water bicycling, using a float belt, is chosen for Roxanna. She is started at the wall to help her learn bicycling and gradually progresses to independent bicycling, making sure she has good trunk control and is secure and independent in this task. Deep-end exercises are added for hip and trunk strengthening. The intensity of these exercises gradually is increased by speeding up the exercise. Her standing exercises and workload are gradually increased by adding resistive equipment to her ankle on the right leg. Gradually, a stepper is added for working on balance and stair climbing strength in waist-deep water.

Roxanna continues to make gains in exercise capability with increased intensity of her workout. She can perform more repetitions for each leg exercise. She can increase the speed of her bicycling movement to increase her aerobic conditioning. Roxanna is seen two times per week for a total of four weeks. At that point, she reports more strength and stability in her trunk and right lower extremity and has less pain with walking. She has become independent with her exercises in the pool and has increased the duration of her workout to 15 minutes of gentle bicycling in the water. At this point, the KT begins to discuss a transitional program and talks with Roxanna about ways she can follow through with an independent water exercise program. She indicates that she really likes the water and also likes the socialization aspect of a class, so an aquatic kinesiotherapy class for those with arthritis is suggested. Such classes are held at the local YMCA, and it is decided that after two more sessions of aquatic therapy she will join the YMCA and continue to maintain the strength and endurance she has gained so far.

Summary

In summary, the healing powers of water are deeply rooted in medical history. In modern day health care, several disciplines have chosen to incorporate the benefits of aquatic kinesiotherapy into their rehabilitation regimen. Kinesiotherapy is one such discipline. In the continuum of care an aquatic KT role most often is in the provision of subacute care, reconditioning exercise, and rehabilitation fitness. As mentioned earlier in this chapter, the role of the aquatic KT will vary based on experience and expertise. Overall, the aquatic kinesiotherapy profession is new and training varies a great deal within and among disciplines. Roles also overlap. Kinesiotherapy is an integral part of the continuum in aquatic therapy.

References

1. American Kinesiotherapy Association. Mission statement. Available from: www.akta.org. Accessed 1998.
2. American Kinesiotherapy Association. Standards. Available from: www.akta.org. Accessed November 9, 1998.
3. American Kinesiotherapy Association. Scope of practice. Available from: www.akta.org. Accessed November 7, 1998.
4. American Kinesiotherapy Association. Our history. Available from: www.akta.org. Accessed July 1, 1999.
5. Corcoran P. Use it or lose it—The hazards of bed rest and inactivity. *Western Journal of Medicine.* 1991;154:536–538.
6. Caudill M. *Managing Pain Before It Manages You.* New York: Guilford Press; 1995:72–73.
7. American Kinesiotherapy Association. Employment and focus. Available from: www.akta.org. Accessed November 7, 1998.
8. American Kinesiotherapy Association. Education and training. Available from: www.akta.org. Accessed November 7, 1998.
9. American Kinesiotherapy Association. Accreditation. Available from: www.akta.org. Accessed 1998.

CHAPTER 9

Massage Therapist

Stacey DeGooyer

Introduction

Massage therapy is the practice or art of using touch to relax and nurture the body, mind, and spirit. Through a variety of techniques, the massage therapist encourages the client's body to function at an optimum level, thus facilitating health and well-being. The physical contact and varying degrees of pressure delivered by the practitioner's hands, knuckles, forearms, elbows, and sometimes feet, combined with judiciously applied body weight and leverage, is designed to create a nurturing, safe, and relaxing sensation. When a client's body lets go of tension and stress, the mental and emotional body can unwind and relax.

The use of therapeutic massage is on the upswing. A 1998 Stanford Center for Research in Disease Prevention (SCRDP) survey cites an increase in the use of massage therapy the preceding year, surpassing chiropractic as the most frequently used provider-based complimentary and alternative medicine (CAM).[1] The study also found that 69% of massage recipients said massage cured or relieved their symptoms considerably. In a 1997 opinion survey released by the American Massage Therapy Association (AMTA), American adults reported receiving three times as many massages in the preceding 12 months than in the previous year.[2] Then, in a 1998 Opinion Research Corporation survey commissioned by the

AMTA, 13% of respondents said they received at least one massage in the previous year, versus 8% in a 1997 survey. Membership in the AMTA has increased threefold to 36,000 members during the 1990s. These trends reflect a rise in the perceived effectiveness and viability of massage.

The professional therapeutic massage community has worked to educate the public and health care professionals to distinguish massage therapy from "adult entertainment" massage and its assumed sexual connotations. Mainstream magazines, including *Life*,[3] *Newsweek*,[4] and *InStyle*,[5] have published articles about the benefits of massage, contributing to its value and legitimacy. Through public awareness and education, massage therapy has matured from a luxurious, pampering spa treatment for the rich to an integral ingredient of health, wellness, and balance for the masses.

More and more health care professionals, such as doctors, chiropractors, dentists, and acupuncturists, are endorsing, encouraging, and even prescribing massage as part their patients' healing regime. As early as 1995, 54% of primary care physicians and family practitioners say they would encourage their patients to pursue massage therapy as a compliment to medical treatment.[6] In San Francisco, the California Pacific Medical Center's Breast Health Center offers complimentary books that recommend massage for women who have had lumpectomies or are undergoing radiation treatments[7] or mastectomies.[8] Often, gynecologists endorse prenatal and postpartum massage.

Medical insurance companies and HMOs are beginning to embrace alternative therapies, offering discounts or full or partial reimbursement for these preventative and rehabilitative sessions. There are three main reasons: the higher cost of conventional medicine, alternative medicine's emphasis on prevention, and acknowledgment of the American public's expenditure on alternative services and products. In 1997, Americans spent an estimated $21.3 billion, including at least $12.2 billion in out-of-pocket expenses on alternative medicine services[9] (including an estimated $4 to $6 billion on massage). The number of plans covering CAM modalities increased from 4 in 1994 to 25 in 1997 to 50 in 1998.[10] Blue Shield of California's Lifepath[SM] Alternative Services Discount Program offers its members a 25% discount on massage when the member chooses a massage therapist from the Lifepath *Health Resource Directory*. In the Stanford study, 22% of respondents said their massage visits were covered by insurance, although the majority of people who see alternative therapy practitioners pay in full themselves. Some hospitals now have massage therapists on site for the patients, caregivers, and employees.

The National Institute of Health opened its Office of Alternative Medicine in 1992 to promote the study and scientific documentation of alternative therapies. This blossoming recognition of alternative therapies has been driving the development of techniques, schools, training, certification, and regulation. Massage, body work, and somatic therapies comprise over 150 techniques. A practitioner often utilizes more than one technique during a session. A few of the more common techniques are briefly described next.

- Swedish or Esalen massage is the most common form of massage in the United States. The practitioner uses specific hand motions, called *effleurage, kneading, friction, petrissage,* and *tapotment,* to push fluids toward the heart. Specific goals include improved relaxation, circulation, and range of motion.[11]
- Shiatsu (finger pressure) is a Japanese acupressure massage. The goal is to improve the flow of energy (*ki* in Japanese and *chi* in Chinese) in the body. Toward this end, the practitioner presses specific points on the meridians or energy pathways, to remove blocks and to free up stagnating energy (ki/chi).[12]
- Sports massage specifically addresses the needs of athletes, both professionals and weekend warriors. Specific muscle groups receive preferential attention, with the goal of preventing injury, improving performance, and decreasing recovery time—whether the client is involved in a competition, an everyday workout, or a zealous training schedule.[11]
- Trigger-point therapy concentrates on identifying tender, sensitive spots in the muscles that can be point specific or radiate pain elsewhere in the body. The therapist locates the hyperirritable spot, often with feedback from the client, then presses or holds the point to release cycles of pain.[13]
- Trager® work, developed by Milton Trager, M.D., utilizes rhythmic rocking movements and stretching to dissolve chronic tension and holding patterns.[14]
- Rolfing®, or structural integration, developed by Ida P. Rolf, Ph.D., focuses on realigning the human structure by deeply attending to overly tight connective tissue or fascia. In a series

and 24 of the 50 states currently have laws requiring some form of licensure, certification, or registration.

Twenty-one states regulate massage, four states have passed laws that are not in effect yet, and one state has regulation in process.[22] State laws supersede local regulations, yet many city and county government agencies do not want to relinquish the regulation of massage. The result is wide discrepancy in the laws, ordinances, rules, and regulations governing massage therapy from one locality to the next.

Where licensing is available, the prevailing trend is toward requiring a 500-hour curriculum. Many professional issues regarding the scope of practice currently are being addressed in the United States. For example, in Louisiana, physical therapists are working to keep licensed massage therapists from performing neuromuscular therapy and other techniques prescribed by a doctor. Under Wisconsin's new registration law, a massage therapist can practice if the terms *massage* or *bodywork* are not used.

Locating a Practitioner

As with most services, for a satisfactory experience, the best way to find a massage practitioner is through referral from family members, friends, or other health care professionals. Directories are available online via the Internet or by calling the state or national offices for a certified or licensed practitioner in good standing. Do not hesitate to ask a prospective practitioner for client and colleague references. Such venues as Harbin Hot Springs in Middletown, California, Two Bunch Palms in Desert Hot Springs, California, and Ten Thousand Waves in Santa Fe, New Mexico, are home bases for aquatic massage techniques, while Whole Life Expose and aquatic therapy conferences are roving ambassadors of water-based massage methods.

The following professional organizations are self-regulating bodies that maintain registries and referral programs. Two are specific to aquatic massage therapy: Worldwide Aquatic Bodywork Association (WABA) and Aquatic Bodywork International (ABI). General massage groups include the American Massage Therapy Association (AMTA), Associated Bodywork & Massage Professionals (ABMP), International Massage Association (IMA), American Oriental Bodywork Therapy Association (AOBTA), and National

Certification Board for Therapeutic Massage and Bodywork (NCBTMB).

Other body work organizations include the American Polarity Therapy Association, Aston-Patterning® Training Association, Association for Hanna Somatic® Education, Hellerwork® Practitioners Association, Feldenkrais® Guild, Reflexology Association, Rolf Institute, Rosen Method® Professionals Association, Touch Pro Institute of Chair Massage, Trager® Institute, and Zero Balancing Association. Contact information for these and other somatic groups can be found in the "Contacts" section of *Massage Magazine* or on the Internet.

Massage Therapy and the Lyton Model

Due to out of pocket expense, low visibility, and the access to pools that are warm enough, aquatic massage therapy has not been fully accessed by the general public. Clients will most likely choose or seek out aquatic massage therapy after trying many other modalities and after a recommendation by another health care practitioner, friend, or relative. Aquatic massage techniques such as Watsu®, WaterDance™, and the Jahara technique are gaining visibility as more and more clients gain exposure. The interdependence of water-based massage therapists on other water-oriented health professionals (see Figure 9–1) will build bridges between the practitioners and aid in the recovery and health of the clients.

Typical Massage Sessions

The main aim of massage therapy is to facilitate an overall sense of well-being. Usually, massage sessions are 55 minutes to an hour of nurturing, caring, relaxing touch. The task of the practitioner is to listen with his or her ears, hands, and heart. Listening includes the careful observance of verbal and nonverbal communication, as well as the kinesthetic cues of tightening and releasing of the client's body and breath. Simply giving one's undivided attention to the physical body is very comforting to the emotional, mental, and spiritual person.

Generally, a session will include a checking-in or verbal intake of how the client is feeling. The practitioner asks if the client would

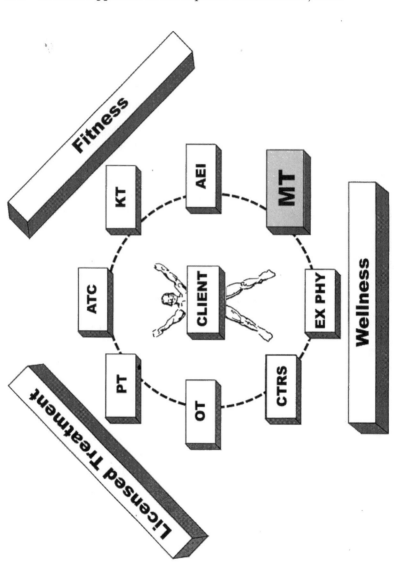

FIGURE 9–1.   Lyton model depicting the massage therapist's role in the aquatic continuum of care.

like the practitioner to focus on any injuries, health concerns, or specific areas of tension. After the client has become comfortable and established in the water, then a moment of connection is taken where the practitioner initially will touch the client, take a few breaths, and be present. Then the practitioner gently introduces movement to the client's body. The pattern or arrangement of movements may be preset in a specific order or series or more intuitive. The structure or randomness depends on the practitioner, the client, and the modality being used. The whole body is addressed, possibly focusing on certain areas needing attention. Then, the practitioner closes a session by smoothly slowing down the vigor of the massage and lightening the contact. A tender finishing hold on the head, shoulders, sternum, or feet will conclude the session. Often the practitioner verbally signals to the client that the massage is over, saying "thank you" and suggesting taking a few moments in the water.

Interaction with Roxanna

The warmth of the water, the suspension that defies gravity in the water, and perhaps even the liquid, waterlike property of the synovial fluid of the joints invite a release of tension in Roxanna's joints. An hour massage offers her simply relaxation and nurturing touch. By increasing circulation to the inflamed areas, stimulating the skin sensors, and arousing endorphin production, massage may help reduce inflammation and pain in the joints. The continual agility and lack of stiffness in the surrounding muscles, tendons, and ligaments are crucial to mobility and quality of life.

The Role of the Massage Therapist in the Continuum of Care

Objective: Facilitate the release of tension in the whole person.

Function: Provide reverent, safe, and caring touch in an environment conducive to relaxation, letting go, and self-acceptance, thereby encouraging the client's own healing mechanisms to work optimally.

20. Dull H. *Watsu®: Freeing the Body in Water*. Middletown, CA: Harbin Springs Publishing; 1993:31–32.
21. Lidell L, Thomas S, Cooke DB, Porter A. *The Book of Massage: The Complete Step-by-Step Guide to Eastern and Western Techniques*. New York: Simon and Schuster; 1984:10–13.
22. U.S. Law and Legislation. *Massage Magazine*. 1999;79:134–135.

CHAPTER 10

Occupational Therapist

Lynette J. Jamison

Daily occupation refers to the activities that individuals engage in during the normal course of a day, including bathing, dressing, eating, working at a job, and in the case of children, playing. The term *occupation*, within the parameters of occupational therapy, refers to the notion of work as treatment. More specifically, it refers to the muscles and mind working together in games, exercise, daily activity, and handicraft. A historical look at "occupation therapy" reveals ancient origins dating back thousands of years ago. Wealthy Egyptians were depicted working in the garden, planting trees and building fish ponds, for peace of mind. The Hebrews and ancient Greeks wrote about the benefits of work on the body and mind. These are two examples of early occupational therapy.[1]

The first signs of occupation therapy in the United States date back to Benjamin Franklin, who established the first hospital in Pennsylvania in 1752. He suggested that inmates who were able should engage in the work task of spinning and carding wool.[1] Idle hands were thought to be the devil's workshop. In the early 1800s, occupation therapy was used to improve social habits of the insane in order to improve the development of appropriate social skills. In 1914, the official name *occupational therapy* was established with significant expansion of the field after World Wars I and II. The first professional school of occupational therapists was established in Chicago in 1915, followed by the establishment of other schools "to furnish forms of occupation to convalescents in long illnesses and to give to patients the therapeutic benefit of activity."[1] These activities met the daily living needs of the wounded soldiers.

Education and Credentials

As of 1999, the American Occupational Therapy Association (AOTA) mandated that an entry-level OT begin at a master's degree level. To obtain a master's degree in occupational therapy, an OT must have earned a bachelor's degree in a related field. The entry-level master's program usually consists of 2–2½ years of core occupational therapy courses. This training encompasses advanced sciences such as anatomy and physiology, neuroanatomy and neurophysiology, kinesiology, physics, and chemistry. Required applied sciences incorporate psychology, sociology, and anthropology. Specific occupational therapy courses consist of critical thinking, which involves analyzing and interpreting evaluative information, learning to establish treatment plans, and learning the different frames of reference, or treatment philosophies. For example, neuro developmental treatment (NDT) is a frame of reference that summarizes an extensive philosophy related to physical and occupational therapy treatment methods and progression. Specific education provides the OT with medical knowledge of disease processes, pathology, etiology, and occupational therapy interventions.

The American Occupational Therapy Association reports over 38 OT schools in the United States. Curriculums focus on psychosocial and physical dysfunction of individuals from infancy to old age with an emphasis on how to learn and solve problems. Aquatic occupational therapy education most often comes after graduation and through independent conferences and courses. Several levels of education exist, from a two-year associate's degree for an occupational therapy assistant (OTA) to an advanced doctorate degree for an occupational therapist (OT). National certification or registration is required for all graduating OTAs and OTs. All states require that OTs and OTAs have initial registration (or certification) by the National Board for Certification in Occupational Therapy (NBCOT). To receive initial registration, the OT or OTA candidate must pass the national registration examination with a minimum of 75% accuracy. In addition to national registration, most states require licensure. Many of the states that require licensure also require registration by the NBCOT for an initial state license. Once a state license has been obtained, continued reregistration by NBCOT may not be necessary.

Medical education for the OT encompasses learning disease pathology and processes, condition and progression of disability, and psychosocial and physical dysfunction. Additional medical instruction consists of splinting, evaluation procedures, treatment planning, administration, and organization.[1]

The OT evaluates patients for cognition, motivation, strength, range of motion, and function in daily activities. Treatment plans are developed from the evaluation data to minimize impairments and optimize client performance. Once treatment plans are established the OT or OTA provides the prescribed treatment.

OTs are known for their work toward improving one's ability to perform daily functions or activities of daily living (ADL), the activities one engages in to complete one's day. ADLs could be as simple as rolling over in bed, using the toilet, dressing, bathing, eating, or in the case of children, playing. Complex ADLs could include installing a computer chip into a computer or designing a bridge. OTs utilize the therapeutic aquatic setting to provide a least restrictive environment. For example, if a client has difficulty performing ADLs due to weakness or inability to move against gravity, placing the person in water diminishes the effects of gravity and supports movement, providing a least restrictive environment. This allows optimal performance of most muscle groups, producing a higher level of ADL execution.[2–5]

Completing a two-year associate's degree and passing the certification examination sponsored by NBCOT with 75% accuracy allows one the opportunity to become a certified occupational therapy assistant (COTA). The OTA curriculum includes applied sciences such as basic anatomy and physiology, neurology, psychology, exercise principles, and adaptive tasks. The OTA learns how to guide a client through exercises and activities of daily living to facilitate optimal independence with life skills. For example, a client who has had a stroke causing left-sided weakness or paralysis often will have impulsive behavior. The OTA may instruct the client to bathe and dress with one hand and emphasize safety skills that may be necessary due to this impulsive behavior. The OTA plays an important role in the rehabilitation process by following through with the plan that the occupational therapist (OT) establishes. The OTA instructs clients in routine exercises and activities as well as guiding them through the rehabilitation process. These services may occur in the water, gym, hospital, or in the home in collaboration with and under the supervision of the OT. Depending on specific state regulations, the OTA may be authorized to upgrade the treatment plan established by the OT and discharge a client from skilled occupational therapy.

Aquatic Occupational Therapy Training

Today few, if any, occupational therapy schools teach aquatic occupational therapy. Registered and licensed occupational therapists and assistants must seek out additional training in this specialty. Local, regional, and national aquatic rehabilitation courses are available. Instruction and national certification are available for Watsu®, the Halliwick method, and the Arthritis Foundation/YMCA aquatic program. Aquatic Feldenkrais® has instruction and a certificate of participation. The following have instruction but no certification: Ai Chi, Bad Ragaz, techniques for neurologic and orthopedic disorders, and diagnosis specific treatment. OTs and OTAs learn water safety from the American Red Cross, YMCA, and Ellis & Associates.[6]

The Roles of the OT and OTA in the Continuum of Care

OTs have been providing aquatic rehabilitation services for over 40 years. In the water, the OT or OTA uses the properties of buoyancy and viscosity to strengthen muscles, improve range of motion, and improve functional performance in activities of daily living. For example, if Susie has lost shoulder function following a mastectomy and is unable to don her blouse, an OT may use the buoyancy of water to increase range of motion and use viscosity to increase strength. The improved range of motion and strength are necessary for donning her blouse. The OT and OTA work in the water to improve daily function and fine motor coordination. When working together with other aquatic disciplines, the OT or OTA enhances patients' functional performance.

There seems to be a significant overlap between physical and occupational therapy, both on land and in the water. Both OTs and PTs have unique skills for determining dysfunction related to daily performance. OTs have special skills for treating upper extremity function, from evaluating fine and gross motor coordination for manipulating buttons, as in donning a blouse, to maneuvering a computer keyboard. OTs are also skilled in treating psychosocial dysfunction when the dysfunction impairs the ability to perform ADLs. OTs are innately different from other rehabilitation practitioners due to the focus on daily function, whether at work or in the home. The OTs' core educational background emphasizes community reentry, work conditioning, and daily performance of self-care. For example, when addressing a patient with fibromyalgia, an OT may utilize Watsu® techniques to address the psychosocial stress level of the client who has difficulty sleeping, which ultimately effects performance of activities of daily living.[2-6]

OTs focus on improving gross and fine motor coordination, as in upper extremity function, specifically to encourage performance of ADLs using such aquatic techniques such as Bad Ragaz, aquatic PNF, and the Halliwick method. Other disciplines may utilize these same techniques to improve leisure skills, functional gait, or for general strengthening. Some OTs have advanced skills to treat psychosocial dysfunction. For example, they may utilize the Watsu® technique to create a sympatholytic response for relaxation or for improved family bonding with clients who have ADL dysfunction due to stress. Other aquatic disciplines, such as physical therapy, may incorporate Watsu® to improve joint range of motion; recreational therapy may use Watsu® for a family leisure activity.[2-6]

Barriers to Provision of Aquatic Occupational Therapy Services

Aquatic occupational therapy is presented with several barriers to providing services, including lack of standardized training, regulation of the aquatic industry, reimbursement, and therapy pools.

Currently no occupational therapy school offers standardized aquatic training. OTs and OTAs who have skill in aquatic occupational therapy developed the skills through weekend workshops and conferences or possibly on the job. With little to no regulation in the aquatic industry, it is difficult to understand who is best suited to provide aquatic service to a given patient with a given problem.[6]

Few hospitals and rehabilitation centers are equipped with warm water therapy pools, making it virtually impossible to provide the much-needed aquatic occupational therapy services. Some facilities that offer aquatic programming do not always have the skilled personnel to provide appropriate services. Finally, a lack of understanding of the value of aquatic occupational therapy and hydrodynamic principles by insurance companies, insurance reviewers, and physicians alike proves to be the single greatest barrier to the provision of aquatic occupational therapy.[4,5]

Reimbursement for aquatic occupational therapy will vary from state to state. States that have strong aquatic occupational therapy programs tend to have liberal reimbursement practices regarding both occupational therapy and physical therapy. For example, in Arizona, occupational and physical therapists have a sound relationship with one of the prominent health maintenance organizations, as do exercise physiologists for cardiac rehabilitation. This HMO offers reimbursement for those therapies but will not reimburse for aquatic recreational therapy or massage therapy. Since each state's licensure regulations and third-party payers vary, investigation is required on the part of an OT or OTA in their particular state regarding reimbursement of aquatic therapy services.[4,5]

OTs and OTAs and the Lyton Model

A patient who enters the Lyton model (Figure 10–1) at the level of aquatic occupational therapy does so via prescription from a physician. Other allied health care professionals often will suggest to the physician that aquatic occupational therapy is indicated for a given patient. After the prescription is received, the occupational therapist completes the evaluation and establishes the treatment plan. Either the OT or OTA follows through with the established plan to reach the established goals.

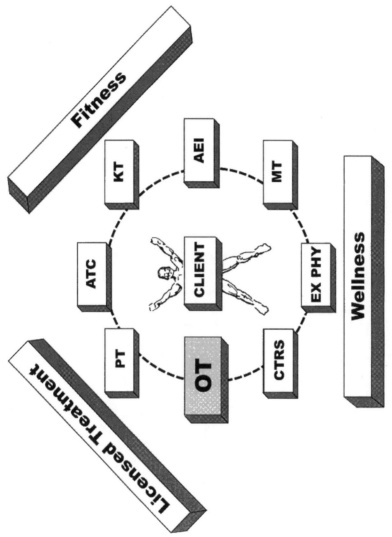

FIGURE 10–1. Lyton model depicting the role of occupational therapy in the aquatic continuum of care.

Interaction with Roxanna

Roxanna is a 64-year-old woman who suffers from a combination of osteoarthritis, rheumatoid arthritis, and obesity. She recently received a right hip replacement. Her surgical site has healed, and her physician has written an order for occupational therapy to evaluate and treat Roxanna. The OT assesses Roxanna's ability to perform activities of daily living, including self-care, ability to perform household chores, and work tasks. It was determined during the evaluation that Roxanna could benefit from aquatic occupational therapy, and a treatment plan was established.

Roxanna has poor flexibility, balance, and body mechanics, making it difficult for her to don her slacks, socks, and shoes. She requires moderate assistance to complete these tasks. Note that she has a 90° hip flexion restriction, as well as no adduction across the midline or internal rotation. She requires maximum assistance with household chores and moderate assistance with preparing meals.

The aquatic occupational therapy plan includes aquatic techniques such as Bad Ragaz and the Halliwick method to improve trunk and upper extremity function by increasing range of motion and strength. These skills are necessary for the movement and balance required to complete the activities of daily living. This will upgrade Roxanna's performance with self-care tasks, household chores, and meal preparation. The aquatic OT or OTA may incorporate turbulence to improve standing balance needed for brushing teeth, combing hair, meal preparation, and work tasks. Aquatic occupational therapy goals are expected to be achieved in two weeks and include

1. Roxanna will don her slacks, socks, and shoes using adaptive techniques and following her total hip precautions.
2. Roxanna will prepare a light meal while standing at the kitchen counter with setup assistance.
3. Roxanna will complete one load of laundry including carrying the load 50 feet, placing it into the washing machine, and retrieving it for drying.

Roxanna will be referred to an exercise physiologist for weight management and to the AFYAP program for continued gains with strength, balance, and flexibility on discharge from occupational therapy.

References

1. Hopkins HL, Smith HD. *Willard and Spackman's Occupational Therapy*, 6th ed. JB Lippincott; 1983:3–23.
2. Johnson C. Aquatic rehabilitation: The unique perspective of occupational therapy. *OT Newsletter.* Autumn 1998.
3. Jamison L. Collaborative differences between occupational and physical therapy, *ARIZOTA Newsletter.* January 1996.
4. Jamison L, Ogden D. Aquatic occupational therapy and physical therapy—do the services really overlap? *OT Practice.* 1996.
5. Ogden D, Jamison L. Aquatic therapy: enhancing rehab through teamwork. *OT Practice.* 1996.
6. Keith L. A survey of the role of occupational therapy in aquatic therapy. Research project. San Jose State University, CA; April 1998.

CHAPTER 11

Physical Therapist

Charlotte O. Norton

Introduction

Physical therapy is a dynamic profession in which its practitioners provide care and services to promote the preservation, development, and restoration of physical function.[1] As a member of the health care team, the physical therapist is challenged to find innovative, effective methods of treatment. In the late 1980s and early 1990s, most new therapeutic facilities included a pool to incorporate an aquatic component to rehabilitation services.

The popularity of aquatic physical therapy has vacillated throughout the years. Promotion occurred during the polio epidemic and after both World Wars and declined with progression in technology.[2] In the 1980s, there was a movement toward a more healthy lifestyle.[2] Life-long participation in activities, including swimming, were encouraged. The aquatic environment provides a safe exercise medium with little risk of injury. Athletes started rehabilitation in the water, and those who were unable to tolerate high impact aerobics used the pool for exercise classes.

Historically, hydrodynamic principles have provided the premise for therapeutic use of water. Research assessing the efficacy of aquatic physical therapy continues to become available, allowing a critical review of outcomes. Because of the increased number of professionals claiming to provide aquatic therapy services, the industry has become muddled in turf battles and confusion. This chapter describes the education, training, and role of the physical therapist (PT) and physical therapist assistant (PTA) in the growing field of aquatics.

Education and Qualifications

PTs are professionally educated at the college or university level and licensed by the state. The Commission on Accreditation in Physical Therapy (CAPTE) has accredited physical therapy education programs since 1960.[1] Prior to 1960, physical therapy programs were approved by various accreditation bodies.[1] As of 2002, CAPTE will accredit only professional educational programs that award post-baccalaureate degrees.[1]

Physical therapy education programs provide the PT with comprehensive knowledge in the basic and applied sciences. The PT treats clients throughout their life span to address acute or chronic dysfunction of movement due to disorders of the musculoskeletal, neurological, cardiopulmonary, and integumentary systems. PTs are trained to use critical thinking skills to bridge theory with practice. The Nagi model[3] for the process of disablement provides physical therapists a conceptual framework to understand the concept of health. This model allows PTs to examine, evaluate, and diagnose clients based on their individual impairments, functional limitations, disabilities, or changes in physical function resulting from injury or disease.[1]

Prevention and wellness activities are a vital part of physical therapy practice. Prevention may be primary, secondary, or tertiary.[1] Primary prevention uses health promotion techniques to prevent disease. Identification of at-risk clients and education about heart disease is primary intervention. Secondary prevention involves decreasing the duration, severity, and consequence of disease through early diagnosis and intervention. The client with diabetes can benefit from an exercise program to promote blood glucose control. Tertiary prevention limits the degree or extent of disability in clients with chronic and irreversible diseases. For example, a client with osteoarthritis can benefit from development of a home exercise program to decrease joint compression, reduce pain, and promote active movement of the joints.

The PT develops a plan of care following a thorough examination and evaluation of the patient. Goals and outcomes are established individually for each patient. Physical therapy services can be delegated to the PTA or other support personnel, such as the KT in a Veteran's Administration hospital or an ATC in an outpatient orthopedic clinic. The PTA is educated and trained to work in conjunction with the PT to provide and monitor the therapeutic program as dictated by state practice acts. The PT is responsible for the actions of the PTA and so should provide direction and supervision of client care.[1]

The PTA is a graduate of an associate's degree program accredited by an agency recognized by CAPTE.[1] The course of study includes one year of general education and science and one year of physical therapy courses including clinical experience. Licensure or registration is not required in all states for PTA to practice. A PTA may modify the physical therapy treatment in accordance with client status within the scope of the established plan of care.[1]

Aquatic Physical Therapy Training

Physical therapy education provides a broad general knowledge base that enables the entry-level PT to treat clients throughout the life span. The field of physical therapy has grown to include a broader knowledge base throughout the years. It has become difficult for practitioners to remain current in all areas of practice, and this has encouraged PTs to become specialized. The American Physical Therapy Association (APTA) recognizes 19 specialty sections for PTs and PTAs to network, learn progressive new approaches to treatment, and share knowledge. Aquatic physical therapy is considered a unique area of practice, as indicated by the development of the aquatic section within the APTA in 1992. Many aquatic PTs treat clients only within their clinical area of expertise such as pediatrics, geriatrics, neurology, orthopedics, or sports medicine.

A study by Morris and Jackson[4] indicated that 60% of bachelor's degree and 67% of master's degeree PT programs and 56% of PTA programs include aquatic physical therapy as a component of entry-level professional education. Knowledge of aquatic physical therapy is acquired primarily in a lecture format. Some programs reportedly teach aquatic physical therapy within other courses, while others offer an entire course as an elective. Most elective courses provide opportunity for students to gain hands-on experience. To address the educational variability, the Aquatic Section of the APTA developed a draft document to clarify the role of the aquatic PT in the aquatic rehabilitation continuum of care.[5]

A PT or PTA can select from a deluge of aquatic physical therapy continuing education courses. National conferences sponsored by APTA address aquatic physical therapy topics such as water safety, reimbursement, and treatment techniques. Weekend seminars provide aquatic continuing education opportunities for PTs and PTAs to learn a variety of treatment options, including Watsu®, Feldenkrais®, Bad Ragaz, Burdenko method, and Ai Chi. The Task Type Training approach and the Halliwick method provide the aquatic physical therapist with a set of principles and guidelines for the application of aquatic treatment. Watsu® and the Halliwick method offer certification on completion of educational requirements. Feldenkrais® requires certification in the land-based method and adaptations are made to use the techniques in the water. The other techniques require no certification for use by the PT or PTA in clinical practice. The Arthritis Foundation and National Multiple Sclerosis Society offer certification courses to teach aquatic exercise classes for people with these diseases.

With the increase of physical therapy treatment occurring in the water, safety is a concern for the patient and the therapist. The Aquatic Physical Therapy Section of the APTA demonstrated its concern for safety by collaborating with Ellis and Associates to develop an aquatic safety course. This course was developed specifically for PT and PTAs who treat patients in the water. The American Red Cross also has a community water safety (CWS) program, which teaches nonswimming, shallow-water rescue skills.

The Role of the PT and PTA in the Continuum of Care

The aquatic physical therapist can use the Nagi disablement model to provide a basis for the application of different treatment techniques to obtain optimal outcomes. The Nagi model describes disease as the process that sets into action the body's defenses and response system. Impairment deals with organic dysfunction (e.g., loss of range of motion or strength). An aquatic physical therapist or assistant can use Watsu®, the Halliwick method, Bad Ragaz, and Ai Chi to treat dysfunction at the impairment level of the classification scheme. An example of an impairment is decreased shoulder range of motion following surgery.

Functional limitation is a client's altered ability to perform a task or activity. Often the properties of water are used to affect functional limitations by making activities, such as walking, easier to complete. A person with back pain may be able to ambulate without an antalgic gait pattern in the water but not on land. This allows for gait training in the pool without pain.

Disability refers to the inability to perform or meet expectations of a role as defined by society. The Halliwick and Task Type Training approaches provide aquatic treatment principles that allow the therapist to deal with disability by integrating functional activities into the rehabilitation process. A patient may have difficulty with independent bed mobility following a stroke. Focusing on vertical and lateral rotations in the water will allow this individual to develop the necessary trunk strength and motor control for independent bed mobility.

PTs set goals to attain functional outcomes. It is imperative that the goals established for aquatic physical therapy are contained in the plan of care for each individual. Impairment level goals may include pain reduction, increased range of motion (ROM), and functional strengthening. Goals addressing a patient's functional limitation or disability may be related to gait training, fitness, or wellness. The ultimate outcome of aquatic physical therapy is to promote optimal function on land. The clarity and precision of treatment to achieve functional outcomes in a timely manner is important to the client and third-party payers.

The primary role of the aquatic PT and PTA is to provide a skilled service throughout the rehabilitation process. This service includes the application of aquatic physical therapy to diminish the effects of impairment and promote the achievement of goals addressing functional limitations. Generally, aquatic physical therapy is reimbursed by third-party payers. PTs and PTAs also have an obligation to provide their clients opportunity for appropriate continuation of their aquatic program. To do this PTs and PTAs must build bridges with the other disciplines involved in the aquatic rehabilitation continuum.

Barriers to the Provision of Aquatic Physical Therapy Services

Barriers facing aquatic PTs and PTAs include lack of third-party reimbursement, professional practice issues, and lack of standardized education. The credibility of aquatic physical therapy and reimbursement for these services present unique challenges for clients. The lack of clear role definition among the multiple disciplines that provide aquatic services creates confusion among consumers and third-party payers.

Fee-for-service reimbursement means that PTs and PTAs work one-on-one with individuals and bill a certain amount for this identified service. Aquatic rehabilitation techniques such as Bad Ragaz and Watsu® require one clinician per client. Managed care in the 1990s has compelled the physical therapy profession to reexamine how therapeutic services are administered. Individualized aquatic physical therapy programs reasonably may be done within a group. For example, a group may consist of two to four individuals, all of whom had a total knee replacement. Their surgical procedure occurred within a four-week period. These clients may benefit from a small group aquatic physical therapy session for peer support while completing individual programs. Often HMOs are willing to pay for this type of service to defray the cost of physical therapy services. Medicare, on the other hand, does not view skilled services provided in a group as reimbursable. Medicare will reimburse for only aquatic physical therapy performed with one PT or PTA working with one client.

One challenging aquatic physical therapy professional practice issue is the lack of clearly defined roles of the aquatic physical therapist and the aquatic occupational therapist. Traditionally, with land-based treatment, the differences have been defined in a variety of ways including upper versus lower extremity or fine versus gross motor skills. The roles often become more confusing when we consider the aquatic medium.

For example, suppose a client is recovering from a recent stroke with hemiparesis affecting the right upper and lower extremities. Most facilities have either a PT, an OT, or an assistant trained to provide skilled aquatic therapy services. If physical therapy is defined as lower extremity and gross motor skills, does this the mean the PT or PTA should not incorporate the patient's upper extremity and fine motor control limitations during the aquatic treatment?

A PT and OT treating the same client may have similar functional outcomes established in the plan of care, but the manner in which the goals are achieved are very different. For example, the patient with right hemiparesis may have an established outcome to live at home with minimal assistance. The PT may establish a goal to increase the patient's dynamic balance for independent ambulation on level surfaces with a narrow-based quad cane. The OT may establish a goal to improve balance to allow the patient to be able to shave and brush his teeth independently while standing at the bathroom sink. Similar confusion exists when examining the roles of other disciplines in the Lyton model. For example, a massage therapist has very different goals for treating a client in the water than the PT. A massage therapist may perform Watsu® with a client to promote relaxation for improving wellness, whereas the PT may use the same technique to promote normal tension or responsiveness in the neuromuscular system to prepare a patient for gait training.

PTs and PTAs and the Lyton Model

A patient may enter the Lyton model (see Figure 11–1) for the aquatic continuum of care via the traditional physician referral. A PT using land-based methods may refer a patient to an aquatic PT for complimentary aquatic physical therapy. It is rare, but an aquatic PT may need to refer a patient to another aquatic PT or OT for a specific aquatic technique he or she is not qualified to perform such as Watsu®. When a patient attains his or her aquatic physical therapy goals, it is often appropriate to refer the client to a wellness or fitness program for continued progression or maintenance of the program. For example, a patient may be referred to a community-based arthritis aquatic program following discharge from physical therapy for a total knee replacement. These programs can be provided by an aquatic PT or PTA who has the appropriate training in group exercise.

As the health care system continues to evolve, reimbursement structures are demanding that physical therapists provide economical services. Physical therapists are forced to depend on other professionals to assist in the care of clients. The relationship of PTs with PTAs, occupational therapists, kinesotherapists, recreational therapists, athletic trainers, massage therapists, exercise physiologists, and aquatic fitness instructors includes communication and sharing

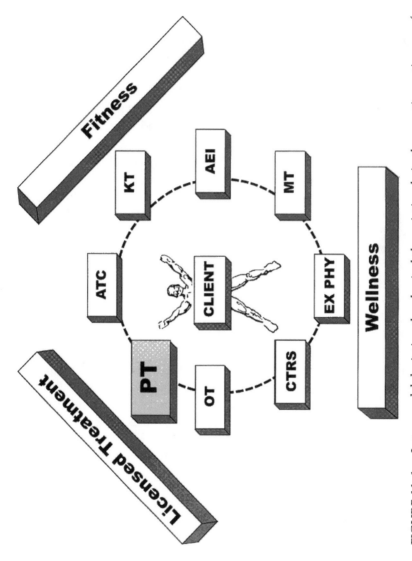

FIGURE 11–1.   Lyton model depicting the physical therapist's role in the aquatic continuum of care.

of information that will allow the continuum of care to be seamless. In an ideal situation, clients should be able to make the transition through a spectrum of aquatic services to enhance their health and well-being with each component having measurable goals for the ultimate outcome. The PT can provide diagnosis-specific information to the rehabilitation team that will allow the clients a safe aquatic experience. When the layers of complexity are stripped away, the reality really is quite simple. The primary role of every aquatic professional is to help clients achieve their health and fitness goals to achieve maximum function.

Interaction with Roxanna

A land-based evaluation can be completed prior to Roxanna's total hip replacement surgery. This would allow the PT to obtain presurgical baseline information and educate Roxanna regarding the surgical procedure and the physical therapy plan of care. She also can be instructed in ambulation with the appropriate assistive device and a therapeutic exercise program can be initiated. Prior to entering aquatic physical therapy, Roxanna's incision should be healed or covered with an occlusive dressing to prevent infection. When she enters the pool, the PT or PTA should complete a safety screening in the pool. Once this has been completed, a plan of care is established to address impairments related to posture, gait, and activities of daily living while observing total hip precautions of no hip flexion past 90°, adduction across the midline, or internal rotation. Functional aquatic physical therapy goals for Roxanna to achieve in two weeks include

1. Roxanna will demonstrate her ability to perform a safe aquatic physical therapy program while observing total hip precautions in one week.
2. Roxanna will ambulate 100 feet in the pool with no assistive device, demonstrating no loss of balance, in two weeks.
3. Roxanna will enter and exit the pool safely and independently in two weeks to allow her to begin participating in AFYAP.

Once Roxanna has met her aquatic physical therapy goals, she will be referred to the the AFYAP program, which can be taught by professionals who attended an Arthritis Foundation training program.

References

1. American Physical Therapy Association. Guide to physical therapist practice. *Physical Therapy.* 1997;77(11):1163–1650.
2. Irion JM. Historical overview of aquatic rehabilitation. In Ruoti RG, Morris DM, Cole AJ, eds. *Aquatic Rehabilitation.* Philadelphia: J.B. Lippincott; 1997:3–13.
3. Guccione AA. Functional assessment. In O'Sullivan SB, Schmitz TJ, eds. *Physical Rehabilitation Assessment and Treatment,* 3rd ed. Philadelphia: F.A. Davis; 1994:193–207.
4. Morris DM, Jackson JR. Academic programs survey: Aquatic physical therapy content in entry-level PT/PTA education. *Aquatic Therapy Report.* 1994;1(4):13–16.
5. Aquatic Physical Therapy Section. *Basic Clinical Competencies Draft 3.* Fairhope, AL: PRADCOM; February 1998.

CHAPTER 12

Certified Therapeutic Recreation Specialist

Fran Coffey Stanat and Ellen Broach

Therapeutic recreation encompasses a continuum of services designed and implemented to enable individuals with disabilities to participate fully in the leisure and recreation aspects of life. The services are functional intervention, leisure education, and recreation participation. While these services often are delivered simultaneously, they will be described separately for purposes of clarity.[1]

Therapeutic Recreation

Functional Intervention

In the first service, functional intervention, the Certified Therapeutic Recreation Specialist (CTRS) provides functional interventions to facilitate improved functional abilities (cognitive, psychosocial, physical, and psychological), health status and/or quality of life.[2] Functional interventions are based on a functional and leisure assessment in combination with activity analysis.[3,4] Functional assessment is conducted to determine physical, cognitive, emotional, and social problems that may be barriers to independent life and leisure functioning. Leisure assessment is conducted to discover leisure abilities and interests, attitudes, barriers, resources, and future leisure directions. Activity analysis is a process of examining the physical, cognitive, emotional, and social skills required for participation in any given activity.[5] Analysis of an activity enables the therapist to determine the feasibility or adaptability of a functional intervention activity for a patient. It also helps the therapist to determine if participation in the activity will enhance patient function.

Leisure Education

When providing the second therapeutic recreation service, leisure education, the CTRS uses teaching and counseling techniques to enable the patient to develop and acquire attitudes, knowledge, and skills to participate in leisure.[6,7] This is an important aspect of treatment because for many individuals with illness and disability employment is no longer an option. Leisure is forced as a way of life rather than as an avocation.[7] For individuals who have spent a lifetime identifying themselves by their employment, adjusting to life where leisure is the prominent theme can be quite devastating. The CTRS can aid the individual to make this transition by exploring with the patient the physical, emotional, cognitive, and social payoffs derived from work. With this information, the CTRS can help the patient choose or continue leisure activities that will enable the same or similar payoffs. The result of exploration in this manner is an individual more likely to find life meaningful which often translates into a person with less reliance on health and human services.

Recreation Participation

Finally, the third therapeutic recreation service, recreation participation is facilitating opportunities for leisure in the least restrictive and most meaningful manner available. Services are generally delivered in community oriented programs that include inclusive recreation services and recreation for individuals with disabilities.[1,8,9] Inclusive recreation refers to ensuring that integrated recreation opportunities are available and accessible for individuals with disabilities.[10]

Recreation for individuals with disabilities refers to programs in the community that are delivered only to individuals with disabilities in a segregated or separate manner. In this case, an individual's disability is so severe that it limits their participation in general recreation programs. This limitation is usually the result of the severity of the disability causing multiple problems for the participant.

The importance of leisure and recreation and the need for the delivery of therapeutic recreation services to individuals with illness and disabilities has been researched. Some of this research has demonstrated that since the inception of the 40-hour workweek, individuals living in contemporary societies will "play" or "recreate" approximately one-third of their lives. If you live to be 75 years old, you will have "played" or "recreated" for 25 years.[10] Other researchers found that in 1998, Americans spent over five hundred billion dollars to participate in wholesome leisure and recreational activities.[11,12] The amount of time and money spent on leisure and recreation suggests that it is an important aspect of life. CTRSs use functional interventions, leisure education, and recreation participation to facilitate maximum access to this part of life for individuals with disabilities. The ultimate goal is to enable individuals to maintain and enhance functional capacity, health status, and quality of life.[11,12]

The benefits of leisure and recreation participation have been studied and identified in terms of personal, social, economic, and environmental outcomes. These outcomes have been categorized into areas that include but are not limited to personal health, human development, social behavior, quality of life, family strength, and reduction in health care costs.[11,12] Research findings clearly indicate that individuals who participate in recreation live longer, more independent lives, free of disease and disability. Further, researchers have discovered that participation in regular recreation enhances the rehabilitation of individuals with physical and psychiatric disorders.[11,12]

The human desires to seek greater challenges, develop more skill, and increase self-awareness of our abilities occurs most often in recreation activities. This correlates with individuals who demonstrate creativity, intellectual ability, and express enjoyment in life.[13] Participation in recreation is essential to a high quality of life. Individuals active in recreation, sports, arts, and culture have greater satisfaction with life, self-esteem, and self-image. Individuals with disabilities also report such participation gives them enhanced self-esteem and self-image as well as increased ability to function independently.[11,12]

Recreation reduces self-destructive and antisocial behavior. Communities with strong youth programs have significantly lower juvenile delinquency rates. Other benefits associated with strong programs include reduction in the incidence of racism, loneliness, isolation, alienation, smoking, and substance abuse.[11,12] Families that play together, stay together.[14] Recreation programs benefit the family and the community with latch key programs, community spirit, and leadership opportunities, creating strong, self-sufficient communities.[11,12] Cost-benefit analysis has found recreation programs associated with lower health care costs. These programs benefit the community by reducing the cost of social service intervention as well as police, justice, and incarceration costs.[11,12] It may be necessary for the community to adapt and modify recreation experiences. The Individuals with Disabilities Education Act (IDEA) mandates that recreation services be provided to enhance educational performance.[15] The Americans with Disabilities Act (ADA) and the Rehabilitation Act were enacted to ensure equal access to public and private recreation in the community.[15]

It is the role of the CTRS to provide functional interventions, leisure education and recreation participation to ensure that individuals with disabilities have the opportunity to take advantage of the benefits of leisure.

Brief History of Therapeutic Recreation

Ancient Egyptian, Greek, Roman, and Chinese cultures all appreciated the value of recreation in the treatment of people who were ill or disabled. Dancing, music, spectator events, drama, exercise, games, and other formalized activities were used to treat, restore, divert, and prevent illness and disability. Much of this humane treatment was lost during the Middle Ages. A *revival of* thoughtful treatment of the ill and disabled that included the notion that recreation could contribute to healing came in the 18th and 19th centuries. Noted people associated with a commitment to the use of recreation for individuals needing habilitation or rehabilitation include Phillipe Pinel, Jean Itard, John Morgan, Dr. Benjamin Rush, and Florence Nightingale.[15] The early work of these leaders put in place recreation staff in many public and private mental health institutions and Veterans Administration hospitals. World Wars I and II saw growth in the field resulting in specialized training for "hospital recreation workers."[8] Accredited college degree programs, from the bachelor's degree through the doctoral degree, are available.

The National Council on Therapeutic Recreation Certification implements, monitors, and maintains a national certification program for certified therapeutic recreation specialists.[15] Two well-established and respected professional organizations, the American Therapeutic Recreation Association and the National Therapeutic Recreation Society, provide educational, technical, and legislative assistance for members of the profession.[10] Therapeutic recreation is practiced in clinical, residential, and community settings. Employment settings include physical rehabilitation facilities, long-term care facilities, mental health agencies, community health and human service agencies, corrections facilities, and home health care. Other employment opportunities are community recreation programs and school systems.[1] Job outlooks place it as the fourteenth fastest growing profession through the year 2005.[16]

Education and Qualifications

CTRSs, at a minimum, are prepared with a bachelor's degree in therapeutic recreation or in recreation with an emphasis in therapeutic recreation. The therapeutic recreation curricula typically include courses required at most major universities with an emphasis in life sciences that includes anatomy and physiology, motor learning, biomechanics human growth, and development. The social sciences include psychology, sociology, and cultural diversity courses. Therapeutic recreation students take foundations courses that introduce leisure theory, health care services, philosophy of practice, ethics, models of therapeutic recreation service, health and wellness, models of professional practice, and management. Knowledge of the etiology, symptoms, and treatment of medical and disabling conditions; psychological reactions to illness and disability; and effects of medications on functioning are examples of other areas required of a therapeutic recreation student. Classroom and field-based courses include assessment skills, treatment planning, and evaluation of patient progress, discharge planning, documentation, activity analysis, and facilitation techniques. Facilitation techniques are interventions that include recreational and educational activities designed to restore, remediate, or rehabilitate function or reduce the effects of disability.

The individual who has completed a degree in therapeutic recreation that incorporates these courses and experiences can apply for certification with the National Council on Therapeutic Recreation Certification.[15] When degree, course work, and field experience credentials have been reviewed and approved, the applicant is eligible to sit for a written examination. Passing this examination allows the individual to use the title certified therapeutic recreation specialist. CTRSs maintain their certification by demonstrating continuing professional development.

Two states—South Carolina and Utah—require therapeutic recreation specialists to be licensed and California has a practice act. A practice act limits the use of the title and job function.

Aquatic Training

Therapeutic recreation students are introduced to aquatic concepts in therapeutic recreation facilitation techniques courses. In addition, most CTRSs receive an introduction to water safety techniques in their professional preparation programs. For many therapeutic recreation students water safety instructor certification or lifeguard training certification may be a college-level requirement. As a result of this additional academic preparation, CTRSs utilize adapted aquatic techniques.

Certified therapeutic recreation specialists receive advanced training in aquatic therapeutic recreation through workshops and conferences sponsored by therapeutic recreation professional organizations or other experts in the field. A certified therapeutic recreation specialist may also acquire additional expertise, on the job, from other therapists skilled in a particular aquatic therapy technique.

The Role of the CTRS in Aquatic Rehabilitation

To explain the delivery of aquatic therapeutic recreation as it relates to the therapeutic recreation model previously described, consider the case of a 35-year-old female with a C-6 level incomplete spinal cord injury who is three weeks post injury and 30% weight bearing on land. In addition to physical weakness, spasticity, and balance problems associated with a new injury, the patient reveals she has enjoyed water activity prior to her injury. She is fearful of the water due to her inability to ambulate and her weak lower extremities. Specifically, the patient reports that prior to her accident, the family participated extensively in water activities that included swimming, boating and fishing. Their real passion, however, was water skiing. The aquatic therapeutic recreation specialist would provide aquatic therapeutic recreation as a functional intervention. Treatment would be delivered utilizing Halliwick, Bad Ragaz, and PNF techniques to improve the physical abilities necessary to restore function as well as continue water activities, especially skiing. The CTRS will also address helping the patient to become comfortable, safe, and independent in the water. The CTRS will use leisure education approaches in combination with aquatic therapeutic recreation to facilitate continued activity in healthy leisure pursuit after discharge. For example, the CTRS would use the adapted water ski in one-to-one treatments in the pool to facilitate improved balance while increasing the patients understanding of adaptive water ski techniques. Due to the recent nature of the patient's injury, she would be unable to learn to ski. One year post discharge the patient would be given the opportunity to learn to ski. A recreation participation service enables the patient to continue this pre-injury leisure pursuit.

The Role of Therapeutic Recreation in the Continuum of Care

The role of the CTRS in the continuum of care is threefold and addresses each component of the TR service model. First, the CTRS provides functional intervention, in the form of aquatic therapeutic recreation to facilitate improved function. During leisure education, the CTRS may use aquatic therapy, adapted aquatics, and/or various aquatic activities such as swimming or aerobics to enable an individual to develop/acquire the attitudes, knowledge, and skills to participate in aquatics as a life-long and life-enhancing activity. Finally, the CTRS may facilitate opportunities for individuals with disabilities to participate in a variety of aquatic activities in the least restricted environment.

Barriers to Provision of Aquatic Therapeutic Recreation Services

Barriers associated with aquatic therapeutic recreation include: referral sources are not aware of the benefits of aquatic therapeutic recreation, limited or restricted physical resources to conduct aquatic therapeutic recreation, payment for aquatic therapeutic recreation services, and the client's inability to continue aquatic activity after discharge from therapeutic recreation services.

First, many physicians and other referral sources are not knowledgeable about the benefits of aquatic therapeutic recreation. Because of this lack of knowledge, aquatic therapeutic recreation is often not recognized, much less utilized, as a treatment modality.

Another barrier to treatment may relate to physical facilities (e.g., therapy pools and tanks). Many rehabilitation hospitals do not have aquatic facilities. Therefore, many CTRSs must utilize community pools for patient rehabilitation. The use of community pools provides an excellent opportunity for community reentry because mobility, public comfort, and problem-solving goals can be accomplished. However, community pool usage poses other problems. These problems include a lack of consistency in treatment if daily transportation is unavailable, water temperature constraints, and flexible programming constraints.

Financial requirements for aquatic therapeutic recreation may provide another barrier. According to Kevin Rath, Health Care Financing and Reimbursement Committee of the National Therapeutic Recreation Society, "Payment for services varies with insurance and managed care companies and how the overall contract is established. An organization in Maine may be approved for aquatic therapeutic recreation by the same company that denied a hospital in Illinois for the same service. Administrators negotiate supplemental or ancillary services in contracts with the insurance and managed care companies that are different. Other forms of reimbursement could be from governmental contracts (state, federal, school district) that the majority of CTRSs do not utilize. Variations in contract or approval for services are with administration, regulators, and state/federal officials. There are different ways organizations bill through other services, room rate, daily rate, per occurrence, or capitation. This may also impact the way the CTRS is reimbursed. Documentation and physician orders also have a huge impact on whether there is advance approval from payers for reimbursement of aquatic therapeutic recreation services. Established programs that have a track record with payers that show cost effective treatment may have a better chance of being approved for this service."[17] Rikki Epstein, Executive Director of the National Therapeutic Recreation Society concurs.[18]

Research supports that a person who is socially and physically inactive is more likely to return for medical services after discharge from rehabilitation.[19,20] Therefore, some companies provide partial reimbursement for client's health maintenance using inexpensive community programs to prevent possible recidivism to inpatient care. No doubt, CTRSs must make services as cost effective as possible. The CTRS's will be able to contribute to the health care provider fabric and most importantly the needs of the patients when all constituencies realize the significance and cost effectiveness of therapeutic recreation services.

Finally, participation in related activities that maintain the benefits of functional intervention services are the pinnacle of aquatic therapeutic recreation. It is unfortunate but true, clients and family may not possess sufficient knowledge or the participant may lack the training or social support to continue the activity after discharge from treatment services. Therefore, an essential consideration in the therapeutic recreation comprehensive approach to aquatic therapeutic recreation is the provision of educational services relative to benefits of using the aquatic environment, aquatic resources, and family training. It is important as part of the therapeutic recreation comprehensive treatment that clients: identify people who could serve as support after aquatic therapeutic recreation treatment, locate facilities providing aquatic interventions, understand and be comfortable with the participation requirements of community-based programs, and be able to articulate and demonstrate a realistic understanding of ability level and needs.

Certified Therapeutic Recreation Specialists and the Lyton Model

The most common method for a client to receive aquatic therapeutic recreation is the traditional medical model of physician referral. Physician referral for aquatic therapeutic recreation is usually based on treatment team information that identifies aquatic therapeutic recreation as the best modality for achieving client therapeutic recreation goals. There are occasions when other therapists may refer or recommend aquatic therapeutic recreation but ultimately the physician writes an order for aquatic therapeutic recreation.

Clients who receive aquatic therapeutic recreation services in community wellness and fitness programs have generally entered the service in one of two manners. First, the CTRS refers clients who have received aquatic therapeutic recreation to community aquatic programs for purposes of maintenance. In other situations, an individual has self-selected aquatics as a health and fitness activity.

Interaction with Roxanna

Roxanna is in continual pain from osteoarthritis and rheumatoid arthritis, has had a total hip replacement necessitated by a fracture, and is overweight (205 pounds, 5 feet tall). Roxanna is able to manage self-care, housework, and shopping. She walks with a noticeable limp and uses a cane for long-distance ambulation. She has been referred to therapeutic recreation for therapy and leisure education, with the ultimate goal of pain reduction, weight loss, and improved mood and self-esteem.

Following a functional and leisure assessment, results indicate that Roxanna lives a very sedentary life, primarily due to her pain. Previously, she enjoyed water aerobics and various craft activities. She feels that the pain and her weight are barriers to leisure participation. She states that she feels tired all the time. The leisure assessment also reveals that Roxanna experiences the depression and self-esteem problems associated with chronic pain. She is also very frustrated by her failed attempts to lose weight. Roxanna is fairly comfortable in the water but has some fears of getting her face wet or losing her balance and not being able to recover. She has noted that, while her pain has not decreased, she seems to have more energy, is in a good mood, and is better able to accomplish tasks after her PT aquatic therapy.

The CTRS's approach will be to introduce two to three additional periods of water activity for Roxanna. Water adjustment and balance activities will be addressed using the Halliwick method. The CTRS will provide Roxanna written information about the benefits of warm water exercise for pain reduction and weight loss. Prior to discharge, the CTRS will implement a community reintegration program for Roxanna, such as an arthritis water exercise program. This two-part program will include helping Roxanna establish personal goals for increased leisure involvement that may lead to pain reduction and weight loss. The second part of the program will be an outing to a community water exercise program where Roxanna is oriented to the facility. The CTRS will suggest modifications if necessary.

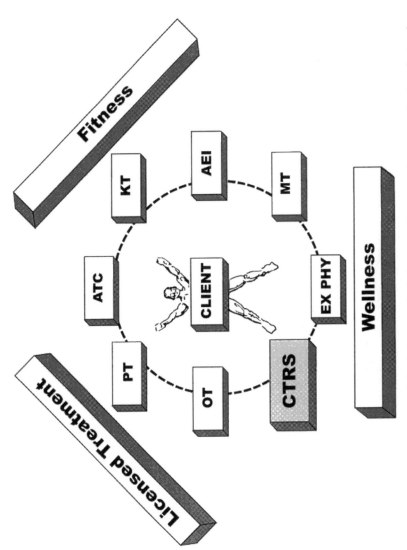

FIGURE 12–1. Lyton model of the certified therapeutic recreation specialist's role in the aquatic continuum of care.

In the case of Roxanna, the CTRS has provided both therapy and leisure education services. The CTRS has also facilitated inclusive recreation opportunities that can enhance functional capacity, health status, and quality of life.

References

1. Peterson CA, Stumbo, N. *Therapeutic Recreation Program Design: Principles and Procedures*, 3rd ed. Englewood Cliffs, NJ: Prentice-Hall; 1999.
2. Coyle P, Kinney W, Riley B, Shank J (eds). *Benefits of Therapeutic Recreation: A Consensus View.* Ravensdale, WA: Idyll Arbor; 1991.
3. Burlingame J, Blaschko T. *Assessment Tools for Recreational Therapy*, 2nd ed. Ravensdale, WA: Idyll Arbor; 1997.
4. Perschbacher R. *Assessment: The Cornerstone of Activity Programs.* State College, PA: Venture Publishing; 1993.
5. Faulkner, R. *Therapeutic Recreation Protocol for Treatment of Substance Addictions.* State College, PA: Venture Publishing; 1991.
6. Mundy J. *Leisure Education: Theory and Practice.* Champaign, IL: Sagamore Publishing; 1998.
7. Dattilo, J. *Leisure Education Program Planning: A Systematic Approach*, 2nd ed. State College, PA: Venture Publishing; 1999.
8. Carter MJ, Van Andel G, Robb G. *Therapeutic Recreation: A Practical Approach*, 2nd ed. Prospect Heights, IL: Waveland Press; 1995.
9. Austin D. *Therapeutic Recreation: Process and Techniques*, 3rd ed. Champaign, IL: Sagamore Publishing, 1997.
10. Chubb, M. *One Third of Our Time? An Introduction to Recreation Behavior and Resources.* New York: Wiley; 1981.
11. Canadian Parks and Recreation Association. *The Benefits Catalogue.* Glouchester, Ontario: Bonanza Printing Copying Centre; 1997.
12. Driver BL, Brown P, Peterson L. *Benefits of Leisure.* State College, PA: Venture Publishing; 1991.
13. Csikszentmihalyi M. *Finding Flow: The Psychology of Engagement with Eveready Life.* New York: Basic Books; 1997.
14. Wilson GT, Enderis D. Milwaukee's "lady of the lighted schoolhouse." *Community Education Journal.* July 1988:16–17.
15. Austin D, Crawford M. *Therapeutic Recreation: An Introduction*, 2nd ed. Needham Heights, MA: Allyn and Bacon; 1996.
16. United States, Superintendent of Documents. *Occupational Outlook Handbook.* Washington, DC: U.S. Government Printing Office; 1998–99.

17. Rath K. National Therapeutic Recreation Society Health Care Financing and Reimbursement Committee. Requested commentary on reimbursement issues in TR; December 1999.
18. Epstein R. Executive Director, National Therapeutic Recreation Society. Requested commentary on reimbursement issues in TR; December 1999.
19. Krause JS, Crewe M. Prediction of long-term survival of persons with spinal cord injuries. *Rehabilitation Psychology.* 1990;32(4): 205–213.
20. Trader B, Rezucka S, Nicholson L. The effects of active recreation participation on adjustment of spinal cord injured patients. Unpublished final report to research review committee. Atlanta: Shepherd Center; 1991.

APPENDIX A

Resources

Aerobics and Fitness Association of America (AFAA)
15250 Ventura Boulevard, Suite 200
Ventura, CA 91403
Phone: 800-446-2322

American College of Sports Medicine (ACSM)
P.O. Box 1440
Indianapolis, IN 46206-1440
Phone: 317-637-9200

American Council on Exercise (ACE)
5820 Oberlin Drive, Suite 102
San Diego, CA 92121
Phone: 619-535-8227
Fax: 619-535-1778

American Kinesiotherapy Association (AKTA)
Plaza Suite 2500
Chicago, IL 60611
Phone: 800-296-AKTA

American Massage Therapy Association (AMTA)
820 Davis Street, Suite 100
Evanston, IL 60201
Phone: 847-864-0123
Fax: 847-864-1178
Website: www.amtamassage.org

American Occupational Therapy Association (AOTA)
4720 Montgomery Lane
P.O. Box 31220
Bethesda, MD 20824-1220
Phone: 800-SAY-AOTA

American Oriental Bodywork Therapy Association (AOBTA)
Laurel Oak Corporate Center
1010 Haddonfield-Berlin Road, Suite 408
Voorhees, NJ 08043
Phone: 856-782-1616
Fax: 856-782-1653
e-mail: AOBTA@prodigy.net

American Physical Therapy Association (APTA)
1111 North Fairfax Street
Alexandria, VA 22314
Phone: 800-999-APTA
Website: www.apta.org

American Red Cross
Contact local chapter office

APTA Aquatic PT Section
323 De La Mare Avenue
Fairhope, AL 36532
Phone: 334-990-8612

Aquatic Bodywork International (ABI)
(formerly the East Bay Watsu® Network)
1406 San Jose Avenue
Alameda, CA 94501
Phone: 510-527-8289

Aquatic Exercise Association (AEA)
P.O. Box 1609
Nokomis, FL 34274-1609
Phone: 961-486-8600
Fax: 961-486-8820
Website: www.aea.wave.com

Aquatic Resources Network (ARN)
1092 West Outer Drive
Oak Ridge, TN 37830
Phone: 423-220-0367
Fax: 423-483-0062
Website: ARNetwork@aol.com

Aquatic Therapy and Rehabilitation
    Institute (ATRI)
Route 1, Box 218
Chassell, MI 49916-9710
Phone: 906-482-9500
Fax: 906-482-4388
E-mail: atri@up.net
Website: www.ATRI.org

Arthritis Foundation
1330 West Peachtree Street
Atlanta, GA 30309
Phone: 800-283-7800
Website: www.arthritis.org

Associated Bodywork and Massage
    Professionals (ABMP)
28677 Buffalo Park Road
Evergreen, CO 80439
Phone: 800-458-ABMP or 303-674-8478
Website: www.abmp.com

Ellis and Associates
3506 Spruce Park Circle
Kingwood, TX 77345
Phone: 800-742-8720 or 281-360-0606

Federation of State Boards
    of Physical Therapy
509 Wythe Street
Alexandria, VA 22314
Phone: 800-200-3031 or 703-229-3100
Website: www.fsbpt.org

International Massage Association (IMA)
92 Main Street
P.O. Drawer 421
Warrenton, VA 20188
Phone: (540) 351-0800
Website: www.imagroup.com

Jahara Technique Central Office
65536 Avenida Barona
Desert Host Springs, CA 92240
Phone: 760-251-9559
Website: www.jahara@juno.com

National Athletic Trainers Association (NATA)
2952 Stemmons Freeway
Dallas, TX 75247
Phone: 800-TRY-NATA
Website: www.nata.org

National Certification Board for Therapeutic Massage
and Bodywork (NCBTMB)
8201 Greensboro Drive, Suite 300
McLean, VA 22102
Phone: 800-296-0664 or 703-610-9015
Fax: 703-610-9005
E-mail: mswiscoski@ncbtmb.com

National Multiple Sclerosis Society
733 Third Avenue
New York, NY 10017-3288
Customer service phone: 212-986-3240
Phone: 800-FIGHT-MS
Website: www.nmss.org

National Therapeutic Recreation Society (NTRS)
22377 Belmont Ridge Road
Ashburn, VA 20148
Phone: 703-858-0784
Fax: 703-858-0794
Website: www.nrpa.org

State Health Department
Contact local number

Worldwide Aquatic Bodywork Association (WABA)
P.O. Box 889
Middletown, CA 95461
Phone: 707-987-3801
Fax: 707-987-9638
e-mail: info@waba.edu
Website: www.waba.edu

YMCA of the United States
101 N. Wacker Drive
Chicago, IL 60606
Phone: 800- 872-9622

APPENDIX B

Glossary

Aid. To provide support, relief, or assistance; to help or facilitate.

Aide. An official or an assistant.

Aquatic or aquatics. Pertaining to water; sports or activities in or on water.

Aquatic rehabilitation. Refers to the use of aquatic activities for the purpose of treatment and education that leads to maximum function, sense of well-being, and a personal satisfying level of independence.

Assistant. A helper; one subordinate to another in rank or function.

Certification. A process by an official body that indicates a person or institution has met certain standards, or person has completed prescribed course of instruction or training. Recognition of level of functioning above basic competency. Also known as *professional achievement*, it implies affirmation of professional status or license to perform specialized skills.

Client. A patient of a health care professional; person receiving benefits or services.

Fitness (physical). Ability to work and have energy for recreational activities; reported to enhance rehabilitation from illness, health, and wellness. Physical fitness-, health-, and skill-related elements of fitness:

Health-related elements include

1. Cardiorespiratory endurance.
2. Body composition.
3. Musculoskeletal flexibility, strength, and endurance.

Skill-related elements include

1. Agility.
2. Balance.
3. Coordination.
4. Speed.
5. Reaction time.
6. Power.

Health. The quality of life involving the total body: physical, mental, emotional, intellectual, spiritual and social components; well-being, not merely the absence of disease or infirmity.

Instructor or instruction. One who instructs, teaches; knowledge of information imparted, the act or practice of teaching, education.

Leader. Guiding or directing head, conductor, or director.

Liability insurance. Insurance covering those who purchase it against losses arising from injury or damage to another person or property.

License or licensure. In the health care professions, granting of official, legal permission to perform medical actions forbidden to be done by persons who are not so licensed. Qualification for license is usually determined by an official body representing the federal or state government. Formal permission from a constituted authority.

Nonlicensed. Having no license, unauthorized, done or undertaken without license or permission.

Participant. A person who partakes, taking part in.

Patient. A person under medical or surgical treatment; one who is sick with or being treated for an illness or injury.

Qualification. Quality or accomplishment that makes a person fit for a function or office.

Recreation. Refreshment by a pastime or agreeable exercise after work; a past time, diversion, exercise, or other resource affording relaxation and enjoyment; to refresh mentally and physically.

Rehabilitation. Process of treatment and education that leads to maximum function, sense of well-being, a personal satisfying level of independence.

Specialist. Physician, nurse, dentist, or other allied health personnel, who has advanced education and training in one clinical area of practice. Conferred when a certifying board exists and the individual has met the criteria for such certification.

Team. Persons associated in a joint action; gather or join in a cooperative effort.

Technician. An individual with knowledge and skill required to carry out specific technical procedures. Person usually has a diploma from a specialized school or an associate degree.

Temperature. Degree of hotness or cold of a substance or body. Temperature is an important part of the therapeutic value of water. Water temperatures for exercise and therapy follow:

Cold: 40–60°
Cool: 60–70°
Tepid: 70–90°
Warm: 90–100°
Hot: 100–110°

Warm for relaxation, warmer to hot for relief of aches, pains, inflammation, swelling, and cooler to cold for stimulation. All temperatures are listed in degrees Fahrenheit. The aquatic instructor teaches in the tepid range.

Therapist. A person credentialed in a therapeutic discipline who utilizes therapeutic activity for the treatment of physical or psychosocial ailments.

Training. Participation in a program of instruction to attain competence in a specific occupation or profession; an organized system of instruction.

Wellness. Integration of physical health to be "well" even in the presence of illness or disease. Reduces the risks of illness and disease, provides satisfaction, control, ability to do more, and take interest in the future.

APPENDIX C

Job Description for Aquatic Exercise Instructor

Modify this basic job description to meet the policies and management structure at your facility.

Position title: Aquatic exercise instructor or aquatic fitness instructor

Description: The aquatic instructor leads class participants through a safe and effective exercise class.

Reports to: Aquatic director

Qualifications
1. High school diploma (minimum).
2. One year's teaching experience (minimum).

Certification
1. CPR certification.
2. First aid.
3. Fitness certification from nationally recognized organization.

Required Competency and Skills
1. Excellent physical health and wellness lifestyle.
2. Excellent instructional and teaching skills.

3. Excellent organizational, communication, and motivational skills.

Requirements

1. Attend four instructor staff meetings per year.
2. Attend continuing education courses or training workshops, minimum of 8 hours total, per employment year.
3. Take community water safety course.

Job Responsibilities

1. The instructor will demonstrate an understanding of the basic principles of exercise physiology.
2. The instructor will be able to identify precautions to prevent an abnormal response during exercise.
3. The instructor will demonstrate ways to modify exercise to improve safety and reduce or increase intensity appropriate for each participant's ability.
4. The instructor will demonstrate an understanding of program design, principles and practices of instruction, and monitoring physical activity (talk test, heart rate, RPE).
5. The instructor will demonstrate an ability to screen participants and identify health problems and risk factors that may require consultation with a physician prior to exercise.
6. The exercise instructor will display professional and ethical behavior in mannerism, attire, speech, and music selection.

Index